INFERTILITY AND INVOLUNTARY CHILDLESSNESS

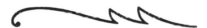

Helping Couples Cope

Beth Cooper-Hilbert, Ph.D.

W.W. NORTON • *NEW YORK* • *LONDON*

To My Guys:
Dad, Gregory, and Joshua
Thanks for your inspiration, support, and understanding

For information about permission to reproduce selections
from this book, write to
Permissions, W. W. Norton & Company, Inc., 500 Fifth Avenue
New York, NY 10110.

Library of Congress Cataloging-in-Publication Data

Cooper-Hilbert, Beth.
   Infertility and involuntary childlessness : helping couples cope /
Beth Cooper-Hilbert.
      p.   cm.
   "A Norton professional book"—
   Includes bibliographical references and index.
   ISBN 0-393-70262-6
   1. Infertility—Psychological aspects.   2. Childlessness—
Psychological aspects.   3. Infertility—Social aspects.   4. Marital
psychotherapy.   I. Title.
   RC889.C64   1988
   616.6'92'0019—dc21   98-24233   CIP

W. W. Norton & Company, Inc., 500 Fifth Avenue, New York, N.Y. 10110
   http://www.wwnorton.com

W. W. Norton & Company Ltd., 10 Coptic Street, London WC1A 1PU

1   2   3   4   5   6   7   8   9   0

CONTENTS

• iii •

ACKNOWLEDGMENTS

WRITING THIS BOOK has been one of the most challenging—and rewarding—experiences of my life. As with all major tasks in my life, I could not have accomplished this enormous undertaking without the support and help of many colleagues, friends, and family.

Much of my inspiration came from my teachers and mentors. Carl Whitaker taught me to challenge the obvious and embrace the absurd, with warmth and humor. Thus I was able to transcend the pain of the infertile couple and create new paradigms for interacting with them. Gus Napier taught me to be patient and to persevere while still engaging my creativity and trusting my intuition. He taught me to enlist the power of the couple system, to mobilize the energy, refocus it, and ride the crest of the wave of change.

Many others guided me, knowingly and unknowingly, throughout this endeavor. Susan McDaniel was most helpful in the initial stages of this effort. She provided my earliest guidance and helped me focus, define, and refine. She was a wonderful source of encouragement and clarification.

I am greatly indebted to Deborah Metzger, who wrote Chapter 1. She readily agreed to my request to contribute the medical aspects of the book. In her tremendously busy life, she found the time for encouragement as well as writing and revising. She always knew the right thing to say in my most frustrated moments; she knew when to promise me that there would be an end to all of this. Debbie was aware of the importance of deadlines and accommodated well, even when her own writing or speaking engagements were quite demanding. She has become a colleague and friend whom I greatly admire.

Many of my friends and colleagues amazed me as they jumped into this chasm with me. They willingly read chapters and were generous with feedback and support. Special thanks to Jeri Hepworth, M. Casey Jacob, and Kathy Laundy, who not only read chapters, faxed them back and forth, but also encouraged me and soothed my tears through many lunches and phone calls. Marilyn Rumsey, who has always been there for me, came through again with much encouragement as well as analysis and comments. Even though she lives far away, her presence was strongly felt. Other significant cheerleaders included Janis Abrahms Spring, who pushed me to keep moving forward and to stay focused when other distractions were more appealing, and my friend Annabelle Howard, whose able guidance and competent writing talents greatly influenced and enhanced my efforts.

Michele Hilbert, a very special person in my family and in my life, gets the award for the most extensive feedback. In her warm, loving manner, she was able to be brutally honest and remind me that's what I asked for—and she was right! I still love her and admire her talents and abilities; and I am grateful for her help.

Karen Zaleski, who was a friend long before I enlisted her expert typing skills, functioned again above and beyond the call of duty. She did her usual perfect job of typing the bibliography. Then, when references needed to be added and deleted "at the midnight hour," she literally accomplished that—while simultaneously packing to leave early the next morning on vacation! Sasha Singer, a librarian at the University of Connecticut Health Center, saved me numerous hours of journal and book searching. She always had patience for my tiresome questions and answered my queries cheerfully and quickly.

Two of the most tireless and creative people, to whom I owe deep gratitude, are my editors: Susan Munro and Regina Dahlgren Ardini. I am appreciative that Susan believed in me: believed in my message and my ability to convey it through the written word. I am so glad she was there to coach me through the initial phases, to normalize much of my anxiety and keep me focused. As I progressed, Regina provided a wonderful calming, steady reinforcement. Somehow she was able to challenge me, force me to clarify my ideas and how I presented them, in a soft, nonthreatening manner. Most often I felt quite empowered, not even realizing I had been challenged. She pushed me until the writing was worthy, and I learned I could trust her to do that. I feel lucky to have had her on my team.

I owe a great deal of thanks to my family. Thanks for putting up with my grumpiness, isolating behaviors, and preoccupation with this undertaking. My husband, Greg, was instrumental in suggesting many of the topic areas and helping me develop my initial outline. His alert, incisive marketing eye helped him realize the significance of many of the topic areas, while his personal sensitivity helped him recognize the importance of this topic—to me as well as to countless others. I am grateful that Greg and my beloved son, Joshua, understood how significant this endeavor has been to me.

INTRODUCTION

MY DAD OFTEN QUOTED the revered Zionist leader Theodore Herzl, who inspired many to pursue the dream of a Jewish state with his vision and invigorating words: "If you will it, it is no dream." Dad believed that with hard work, difficult objectives could be achieved. Certainly this has been true in most of my life experiences. If I tried hard enough, I could accomplish the sought-after goal.

What shocked me—and what I had to teach my dad—was the enormity of an insurmountable obstacle called infertility. There was no "willing" it to be different. There was no "just being smart enough."

Infertility is the crisis of the '90s. It affects one in six couples— over ten million people. It is a medical, psychological, and social problem. The technology employed in infertility treatments is big business. Medical intervention offers hope, but it is expensive and complex, exacerbating the stress couples feel. Further, such sophisticated medical technology has begun to change the way families are defined in our society.

Gender differences are accentuated under the stress of infertility. Most find it at least as stressful as divorce or the death of a close family member. The crisis is severe and enduring and may persist for years. Many will be equally distressed by an inability to have a second or third child as others are by an inability to have their first.

Families are often torn apart as rivalries and jealousies fester. One sister may resent the other's pregnancy, thus refusing to attend a family function. Holidays, usually times of family gatherings and closeness, may become aversive for the infertile couple, who dread being around young children or new babies.

Since infertility is such a highly prevalent crisis, mental health practitioners need knowledge of the medical and psychological aspects associated with the issue. They must appreciate the enduring nature of infertility, which is seldom resolved through medical intervention alone. Most importantly, clinicians need to understand the systemic reverberations of infertility: It affects every member of the family, not just the infertile couple and the yearning future grandparents. Clinicians must also recognize that couples and families will often emphasize other issues when they come for therapy. Most often clients are unaware of the pervasive and enduring impact of their infertility. Couples may report poor communication or a lack of meaning in their lives. Families may ask for help with a depressed member or an acting-out child, not realizing the child is merely reacting to the parents' unresolved infertility. The unfinished issues may result in overprotectiveness, resentments, or parental depression. Clinicians need to be alert to these hidden aspects of infertility and know how such issues might impact the couple or family. Further, they must know how to successfully help couples and families finally resolve their infertility experiences.

Variant family forms, singles, gay and lesbian couples, and blended families present special considerations around their infertility resolution. Familiarity with and understanding of these considerations are important for the clinician encountering this vastly growing population.

Charting Your Course: A Guide to the Contents

Chapter 1: A Physician's Perspective

Working with the infertile couple involves being familiar with medical as well as psychological issues. Chapter 1 explains the male and female biology, problems that may be related to an individual's biology, the diagnostic procedures, and the medical technology. It is essential to have an understanding and knowledge of what the couple is experiencing medically in order to address their emotional reactions. The couple may also need help confronting a change of course, whether that involves trying a different procedure or struggling with a decision to end treatment.

Chapter 2: The Couple's Developmental Cycle

When working with these couples, it is important that infertility be viewed as a couple's dilemma and that intervention involve both partners—the couple *system*. Chapter 2 provides the context for viewing the couple as a system that must be recognized and worked with as the focus of treatment. The chapter reviews the partners' stages of development as they struggle to integrate their singular lives into a couplehood. As they traverse together through life, they experience developmental milestones as individuals and as a couple. They struggle to define a comfortable level of involvement with their families of origin, to establish holiday rituals, determine how to handle money, and find the meaning or place for children in their lives. Then, when the unanticipated crisis of infertility confronts them, they must deal with the shock and disappointment. Therapists must learn the tools that can help the couple system continue to grow and develop as the partners face infertility and work to resolve it.

Chapter 3: The Emotional Stages of the Infertility Crisis

Chapter 3 provides a map through the emotional stages of the infertility crisis. The many losses experienced by infertile couples are similar to the grief and loss stages described by Kübler-Ross (1969). As the couple navigates through the stages, there are profound effects on the marital system, such as intense conflict, sexual difficulties, and constricted communication. The clinician needs to know how to respond as the couple experiences the initial shock, often followed by denial, anger, and grief. As the partners move toward resolution, they need direction, support, and clarification from a therapist who comprehends their experience. When a biological child is unlikely or impossible, the couple needs someone knowledgeable enough to push them to let go and move on. Since there is no cure for infertility even if eventual pregnancy is achieved, couples need to discover some kind of peace and resolution. This chapter discusses the stages of therapeutic intervention and gives specific instruction for the therapist.

Chapter 4: The Impact of Gender in Dealing with Infertility Issues

While husbands and wives both experience significant stress when confronted with difficulty in achieving pregnancy, there are differences in how they express the stress and cope with it. For example, husbands frequently report feeling helpless with their wife's distress and reluctant to express their own. Thus, they often withdraw, which their wives may interpret as an indication that they don't care. Wives may communicate more freely their disappointment and anguish, but need parameters around their expression because such emotion can consume the couple's time and energy and can be overwhelming to the husband. Chapter 4 discusses these gender differences and methods of helping the partners bridge them.

Chapter 5: Struggling with Infertility: The Context of Religious and Cultural Paradigms

Family and children signify varied meanings in different cultures. The advent of children in most couples' lives signifies the rite of passage into adulthood. It serves as a link and a bond between generations. When there are religious or cultural differences within the couple system, infertility may present an entire set of additional stressors. Chapter 5 discusses multicultural considerations within the context of infertility. Religious differences may make one partner feel he or she is being punished for marrying outside his religion. Cultural differences may create similar guilt and provoke real or perceived pressures from extended family members to seek a new partner to carry on the lineage. The infertility experience may magnify religious or cultural differences and put further pressures on the couple. The therapist must be sensitive to such issues and how they affect the couple's ability to deal with the infertility crisis.

The therapist also must be versed in intervention techniques that will best address religious, ethnic, or cultural differences.

Chapter 6: When Infertility is Not the Presenting Complaint: Using Genograms to Explore the Issues

Often, couples present for therapy without any conscious knowledge that their unresolved infertility issues underlie their present complaints. There may be communication difficulties left from the times it was too painful to talk about the future, or the times one or both could only communicate about the pregnancy that wasn't occurring. Depression or listlessness may be the result of unresolved grief. Sometimes the couple presents with anger or explosiveness that is more intense than any recent precipitant warrants. If the couple has children, by whatever means, the partners may be overprotective or overinvolved. Chapter 6 discusses how the therapist can recognize that infertility is the problem when it is not the presenting complaint. The clinician is guided in the use of the genogram and other intervention strategies to help identify these couples or individuals and help them resolve their infertility or grieve their loss in order to achieve more effective functioning.

Chapter 7: Involuntarily Childless But Not Necessarily Infertile

There are other segments of the population who are not necessarily infertile, but who are involuntarily childless nonetheless. Singles and gay and lesbian couples may not be infertile, but they experience much of the same pain, loss, and grief as the infertile. Spouses in blended family configurations may not be infertile, but they may be involuntarily childless. A childless man or woman may marry someone who already has children and does not wish more. Or a woman may marry for the first time when she is already beyond her childbearing years. Even if she wishes to consider a donor egg procedure or adoption, her new spouse may be opposed. Some individuals may have coupled later in life and feel a biological pressure to decide and act on childbearing when they are not psychologically or developmentally ready as a couple. These out-of-phase couples require specialized therapeutic approaches that are sensitive to their issues. Chapter 7 focuses on those who are involuntarily childless, the options available to them, the ramifications of these options, and ways to work with these variant family forms.

Chapter 8: The Implications of Biotechnology for the Family and the Culture

The final chapter discusses the far-reaching implications that the new reproductive technologies have created for the family and the culture. Biotechnology and genetic engineering have forced us to redefine the family. We now have biological parents and rearing parents. A child's aunt may also be her biological mother. Since fertilization can take place outside the body using a family member or a stranger's donated egg or sperm, we are encountering new ways of creating families, new family permutations. This chapter also emphasizes the need for social awareness, medical ethics, and legal action to keep pace with this complex technology.

"If You Will It, It Is No Dream"

In a sense, writing this book has been the fulfillment of a dream. It has been a healing, a bridging of life experience and yearnings of the heart with vast clinical experience. It has been a way to move from the surreal to the real: from the devastation created by one of nature's cruelist tricks, infertility, to the generation of one of the most potent healing methods, telling the story. It has been a journey from hopelessness and powerlessness to joy and elation through new forms of creativeness.

Dad always pushed me to strive for the next hurdle. He planted the seeds that ultimately blossomed into the energy and motivation to problem-solve and move forward. No one can anticipate the trials that may confront us in our lives. As mentors or parents, we can only hope we have planted our gardens well and that our seedlings will have enough strength and fortitude to weather the storms. Thanks, Dad, for the inspiration and courage to help me survive my infertile times. Out of my difficulties I hope I have been able to create a fertile path for other suffering souls to travel. I hope my experience and my knowledge will make others' burdens more solvable.

I have had many excellent and well-known mentors in my life. I am grateful for all they have imparted, even when it was difficult to hear. However, the most challenging mentor has been life itself, from which no one can really escape, but from which we all learn the most arduous and painful lessons. I hope I have in some way helped those who wish to help and paved for them a more comfortable and enlightened path, as a good parent, mentor, and therapist should.

1
A PHYSICIAN'S PERSPECTIVE
Deborah A. Metzger

> Infertility patients are not sick but they are heart sick, and the
> help they seek is to them as urgent as any in medical practice.
> —Dr. Sophia Keegman

MOST COUPLES ASSUME that they will become pregnant when they wish, that once they stop using birth control, pregnancy will happen right away. Although this occurs without too much difficulty for the majority of couples, others soon realize that conceiving is not as easy as they anticipated. At some point in their lives, at least 15 percent of couples will experience some degree of infertility (Speroff, Glass, & Kase, 1994) with all of its accompanying feelings and frustrations.

From a purely medical perspective, infertility is defined as the inability to conceive after 12 months of regular, unprotected intercourse or the inability to carry a pregnancy to live birth (Speroff et al., 1994). However, for most couples, infertility is more than just a physical condition. Infertility represents a seemingly insoluble problem that taxes them physically, financially, and emotionally. Therefore, it is no wonder that emotional problems and infertility often occur together. The angst of dealing with the emotional issues of infertility is often compounded by the stress involved in undergoing infertility evaluation and treatment. The therapist who treats infertile partners or couples will be better prepared to provide optimal support when he or she understands the medical issues involved in treating infertility.

The Reproductive System

In order to understand infertility, it is necessary to understand the normal process of reproduction, which culminates in the successful merging of the sperm and egg and the creation of a unique individual.

A woman's reproductive cycle is determined by the cyclic interaction of her hypothalamus, pituitary, ovaries, and uterine lining (endometrium) (Figure 1.1). The hypothalamus releases gonadotropin-releasing hormone (GnRH) approximately every 90 minutes. Follicle stimulating hormone (FSH), released by the pituitary

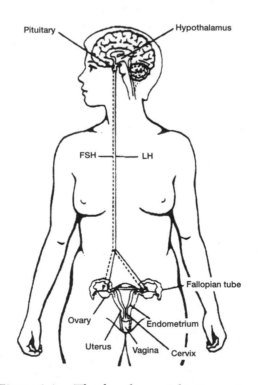

Figure 1.1. The female reproductive system.

in response to GnRH, begins the 28-day reproductive cycle at the time of menstruation (day 1 of the cycle) by initiating egg maturation in the ovary. Although approximately 20 eggs may start this process each month, only one egg usually survives. The mature egg(s) is released in response to a surge of luteinizing hormone (LH), which occurs approximately 14 days after the beginning of a menstrual period. Once released from the ovary where maturation has taken place, the egg begins its journey by entering the fallopian tube, where, if intercourse has taken place in the last 48 to 72 hours, there may be sperm. In order for fertilization to occur, the sperm must be able to penetrate the outer shell of the egg (zona pelucida). The fertilized egg continues its journey through the fallopian tube, during which cell division and early differentiation begin, resulting in formation of a blastocyst. By day 20 to 24, the blastocyst arrives in the uterine cavity and implants in the endometrium, which has been prepared by estrogen and progesterone secreted by the ovary (Figure 1.2). If implantation occurs, the blastocyst produces human chorionic gonadotropin (hCG), which prolongs the secretion of estrogen and progesterone from the ovary until

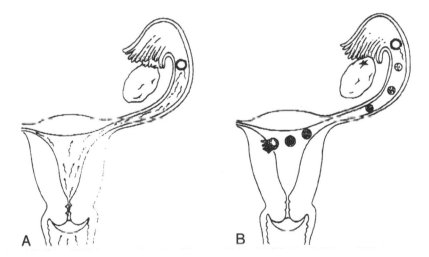

Figure 1.2. *Process of conception. A: The sperm enters the female reproductive tract and fertilizes the egg in the fallopian tube. B: The fertilized egg undergoes cell division in the fallopian tube on its way to the uterus, where hopefully it will implant.*

the placenta is developed sufficiently to take over this function. If fertilization or implantation fails to take place, the ovary "automatically" stops production of estrogen and progesterone, causing the prepared endometrium to be cast off as menstrual flow.

There are several aspects of the male reproductive system that are analogous to the female reproductive system. Testosterone and sperm production are regulated by LH and FSH produced by the pituitary gland in response to GnRH secretion by the hypothalamus. Unlike the female reproductive system, there is no cyclicity and instead of production of 400 eggs during the reproductive years, the male produces millions of sperm until death. The entire process of spermatogenesis (Figure 1.3) takes place in the testicle, where conditions are generally optimal for sperm production: a temperature 2°C lower than the core body temperature and a barrier between the blood and the testis (to prevent the production of sperm antibodies). The sperm move gradually from the testis to the epididymis, an organ that stores and nourishes them as they mature. Once sperm are completely mature, they move into the

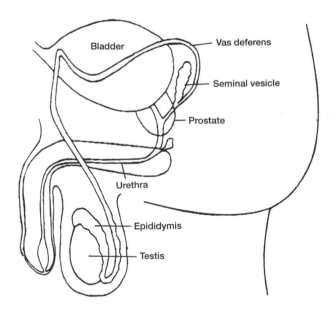

Figure 1.3. The male reproductive system.

vas deferens. This tubal structure connects the epididymis with the seminal vesicles, the two pouchlike glands that provide storage for the mature sperm. The entire process of spermatogenesis from cell division to sperm maturation takes about 72 days. Just prior to ejaculation, sperm from the seminal vesicles combine with a thick fluid from the prostate gland to create the semen, which may then be deposited in the vagina.

The earliest stages of spermatogenesis are easily influenced by fever, prolonged exposure to heat, and chemical exposure. Thus, suboptimal sperm will be ejaculated for two to three months following exposure to these conditions. Likewise, any fertility treatment directed toward the male may take three to four months to become apparent in the semen analysis. Sperm counts drop with frequent ejaculation and may rise with two to seven days of abstinence. Longer periods between ejaculations may result in a drop in sperm quality. Generally, these variations in the quality of semen have no demonstrable effect on the fertile population, but they may contribute to infertility in those having trouble conceiving.

Causes of Infertility

More than 1 in 12 couples in the United States has difficulty conceiving (Mosher, 1988) and it may be as high as 1 in 7 for couples in their late thirties and early forties (Stovall, Tomah, Hammond, & Talbert, 1991). We are in the midst of an infertility epidemic, the unforeseen consequence of several socioeconomic trends. The advent of reliable contraception, the women's movement, and an economy that pushed women into the workplace during their most fertile years led many couples to wait to have children so that the fertile period may have passed them by. As a woman ages, it is harder for her to get pregnant and to stay pregnant. This appears to be a direct consequence of an age-related decline in her ovarian endowment, which results in a decrease in total number of eggs and egg quality. In addition, the sexual revolution has resulted in a sharp rise in sexually transmitted diseases, which can impair fertility. Awareness of these issues causes many couples to experience intense guilt over past "mistakes," such as therapeutic abortions, adoption, sexually transmitted diseases, and promiscuity.

Considering the precision and intricacy with which the human reproductive system functions, it seems miraculous that babies are conceived and born without difficulty to the majority of couples. On the other hand, conception is ensured by the excesses of nature in providing over 400 ovulations during the lifetime of an average fertile woman as well as millions of sperm in a single ejaculate of a fertile man. However, any change in this complicated sequence of events can result in infertility. In order for conception to occur, sufficient numbers of normal, motile sperm must be able to reach the fallopian tubes, a ripe egg has to be released, and the uterine lining must be appropriately prepared to accept the fertilized egg. Forty percent of infertility can be attributed to male factors and the remainder to female or couple factors (Healy, Trounson, & Andersen, 1994). The vast majority of these problems are treatable, which can be attributed to the tremendous strides in the diagnosis and treatment of infertility. About 65 percent of the couples who seek medical help eventually succeed in having children (Speroff et al., 1994). The most common causes of infertility are listed in table 1.1.

Stress and Reproduction

It comes as little surprise that stress and infertility are associated. Although this implies a cause and effect relationship, it appears that the emotional problems that confront the infertile couple are more often the result of, rather than a cause of, infertility. Regardless of the source of the stress, there is ample evidence that chronic stress can adversely affect reproductive function. The gradual unraveling of the complexities of neuroendocrinology have allowed a greater understanding of the role that stress might play in infertility. Catecholamines, prolactin, adrenal steroids, endorphins, and serotonin, which mediate different aspects of the "fight or flight" response, affect all aspects of male and female reproduction.

Awareness of the intense, often overwhelming, emotional turmoil that infertile couples face places the therapist in a critical role in the enhancement of the emotional well-being of the couple and

TABLE 1.1. CAUSES OF INFERTILITY*

Abnormal sperm motility (asthenospermia)

Adhesions (scar tissue) from previous surgery or pelvic infections

Antisperm antibodies (in either partner)

Blocked fallopian tubes (tubal obstruction)

Cervical mucus that does not allow the sperm to enter the uterus and fallopian tubes (cervical factor)

Endometriosis

Hormonal abnormalities (hyperprolactinemia, hypo- or hyperthyroidism or adrenal hormone abnormalities)

Irregular ovulation or failure to release an egg (anovulation)

Maternal age >35

Repetitive miscarriage

Retrograde ejaculation

Suboptimal sperm or lack of sperm (oliogspermia or azoospermia)

Unexplained infertility

Uterine lining which is inadequately prepared (luteal phase defect)

*Listed alphabetically. Note that a single cause of infertility is rarely found; more than one of these factors in either or both partners may contribute to conception difficulty.

in the fertility potential as well. Thus, the role of the therapist may be as critical in achieving a pregnancy as the fertility treatments prescribed by the physician.

Stress can manifest itself in a variety of ways. Couples with an otherwise good relationship may develop signs of marital discord and those with normal sexual function prior to their infertility problem may develop decreased frequency of intercourse, orgasmic dysfunction, midcycle male impotence, or vaginisimus. Because conception and infertility diagnostic testing may require precise timing of intercourse, many couples can experience loss of sexual spontaneity. Intercourse becomes a "chore." As a result, there may be discomfort during intercourse due to decreased lubrication in the woman or impotence in the man. An occasional episode of impotence or lack of desire is common for couples experiencing infertility. Persistent problems indicate the need to consult with a health care provider or therapist.

In females, emotional stress and menstrual disorders have been associated since ancient times. The local secretion of biogenic amines and endogenous opioids, as well as the production of catecholamines from the adrenal gland, are altered with stress and upset both the delicate regulation of the hypothalamic pulse generator and the release of gonadotropins from the pituitary. The resulting "domino effect" is sufficient to upset the entire reproductive process, resulting in amenorrhea, irregular menstruation, or luteal phase inadequacy.

The function of the reproductive organs is regulated in part by sympathetic and parasympathetic nerves. Thus, the over- or underfunctioning of these nerves may explain mechanisms through which emotional stress might directly affect ovulation, uterotubal function, or pregnancy maintenance. Alteration in neurotransmitter release from sympathetic and parasympathetic neurons has been demonstrated to cause alterations in egg release, transport of the egg or embryo by the fallopian tube, and production of estrogen and progesterone from the ovary, thus contributing to decreased fertility.

Emotional factors may also negatively affect fertility in the male. Spermatogenesis has been found to be profoundly suppressed in incarcerated men who have been sentenced to death. In infertile men undergoing in vitro fertilization (IVF), semen quality deteriorates significantly during the interval between the pre-IVF evaluation and the sample used to inseminate the eggs after retrieval (Harrison, Callan, & Hennessey, 1987; Kemeter, 1988).

Physiologic explanations for these observations can be made on the basis of several experimental observations. For example, administration of supraphysiological levels of intravenous epinephrine to healthy men leads to significant reduction in testosterone production. Similarly, high levels of epinephrine and corticosteroids secreted by the adrenal glands can influence the cerebral cortex, hypothalamus, pituitary, or the testicles. Four types of disturbances in reproductive function that are directly related to emotional stress have been reported in men: impotence, sham ejaculation, retrograde ejaculation, and oligospermia (Seibel & Taymor, 1987).

Infertility Evaluation

Although approximately 15 to 20 percent of couples desiring a pregnancy have difficulty conceiving, less than half seek help from a health care provider (Healy et al., 1994). For the couple having trouble conceiving, the best opportunity for evaluation and treatment is with a physician who has a special interest and expertise in infertility. Evaluation and treatment can be handled initially by a primary care physician, obstetrician/gynecologist, or urologist. However, for longstanding infertility (>2 years), lack of conception after short-term standard treatment, or when the woman is over 35 years of age, a fellowship-trained infertility specialist, who can offer the full breadth of infertility treatment, should be consulted.

Identifying fertility problems involves performing a variety of tests to determine the problem and/or to determine the most appropriate treatment regimen. The general rule followed by most physicians when performing an infertility evaluation is to begin with the simplest and least invasive tests. There may be considerable variation among physicians in their approach, depending on their level of training in infertility. If the cause of infertility is not identified from these tests, more involved testing may be required. Both partners should be evaluated simultaneously, since limiting the evaluation to one member of a couple can delay or prevent a complete understanding of why a couple isn't conceiving.

The first step in evaluating infertility is to perform a detailed medical and personal history. This includes information from the couple about past medical and surgical history, current health status, occupational risks, history of sexual development, previous use of birth control, past gynecological and obstetric history, and current sexual practices. Although the vast majority of ob/gyns and infertility specialists have been trained to focus on treating women only, both partners should be examined. The male exam is generally deferred unless an abnormality is detected in the semen analysis, at which time he is referred to a urologist. At the time of the wife's physical exam, secretions from the cervix are tested for the presence of chlamydia and gonorrhea and the pelvic organs are palpated for evidence of abnormalities.

Four areas are assessed by the infertility evaluation, which encompass different aspects of the reproductive process: the number and quality of sperm, maturation and release of an egg, barriers to fertilization, and barriers to implantation and maintenance of pregnancy. The testing, which attempts to determine if problems exist, is discussed in more detail in the sections that follow.

The Number and Quality of Sperm

The semen analysis is the single most important test in the evaluation of the male. It provides information about a number of factors related to fertility, such as volume of semen, number of live sperm, sperm motility, and sperm morphology. In order to perform the test, a semen sample is collected by masturbation into a sterile container provided by the physician. If obtained at home, the sample must arrive at the lab within one hour of collection. Men are also given the option of collecting the semen sample in the office, but appropriate facilities are often limited to an exam room (sometimes without a lock!), public restroom, or "other" type of room. The wives may be encouraged to "participate," although these instructions are often omitted depending on the comfort level and sensitivity of the health care provider.

In spite of the fact that the semen analysis is noninvasive and involves a "natural" process, most men are more or less reluctant to have the testing performed. There are several issues that contribute to this ambivalence. First, a man may fear that he will be found "lacking" or "inadequate" on the basis of the numbers from the semen analysis. Second, he may worry that he may be the cause of the couple's infertility. And finally, there are cultural pressures regarding the "unmanliness" of masturbation compared to sexual intercourse.

Maturation and Release of an Egg

Blood tests may be performed to detect abnormalities in a variety of hormones related to reproductive function such as prolactin and thyroid hormones. In addition, women over the age of 35 may also undergo assessment of day 3 FSH and estradiol (Muasher et al., 1988; Scott et al., 1989). These levels determine how hard the pituitary must work to stimulate the ovary and thus indicate if there is a declining supply of eggs.

Basal body temperature (BBT) charting continues to be an inexpensive and informative indicator of ovulation and can be helpful for the scheduling and interpretation of tests. In order to chart her temperature, a woman must take her oral or vaginal temperature every morning before arising and plot the temperature on a graph. The temperature remains low until ovulation occurs, at which point the temperature rises by approximately one degree Fahrenheit. Unfortunately, ovulation can only be determined retrospectively, making determination of the fertile time a guessing game. Many infertile women who come into an infertility specialist's office with months of temperature charts are visibly relieved when informed that these charts are no longer necessary. In recent years, urinary LH testing kits (ovulation predictor kits) have been developed to determine the approximate time of ovulation 24 to 48 hours in advance. This method is more helpful than BBT charting in planning intercourse around a woman's most fertile days and for scheduling other tests and procedures.

Barriers to Fertilization

In order for conception to take place, the sperm must be able to penetrate the cervical mucus and the fallopian tubes must not have any interruptions. To determine if the uterine cavity is of normal shape and if the fallopian tubes are open, a radiological test known as an hysterosalpingogram (HSG) is performed. The test is performed after a menstrual period but before ovulation and takes place in a radiology facility. The woman is asked to assume the lithotomy position (knees bent and legs spread apart) to allow insertion of a speculum. A tenaculum is attached to the cervix and a narrow tube is introduced into the cervical canal through which dye is injected. It is not unusual for the woman to feel intense cramping during the procedure unless local anesthetic is injected just prior to the dye. X-rays are taken of the image of the dye within the uterus and tubes.

The postcoital test assesses the quality and consistency of the cervical mucus and must be performed a day or two prior to the expected time of ovulation. For most of the month, the woman's cervix produces a barrier of thick mucus that prevents the entry of bacteria, sperm, and other organisms into the uterine cavity.

Just prior to ovulation, the cervical mucus changes consistency under the influence of rising levels of estradiol, allowing sperm to enter. In order to determine if the cervical mucus is interfering with conception, the couple is instructed to have intercourse prior to an appointment with the physician. The cervical mucus is then examined for quantity and consistency as well as the presence or absence of motile sperm. This testing can be stressful for a variety of reasons. One reason is that physicians vary in their instructions to the couple regarding the amount of time between intercourse and examination. Some physicians want to perform the test within 1 to 2 hours of intercourse, while others feel that 12 to 18 hours is more indicative of natural conditions. When both partners work and the test is to be performed within 1 to 2 hours, intercourse during the workday can require some creative planning, such as meeting in a motel, rushing through traffic to rendezvous at home, or attempting to overcome situational impotence. It's no wonder that couples sometimes require two or three cycles in order to be able to have the test performed!

Many women with scar tissue or endometriosis may not have any indication by symptoms, examination, or testing that these infertility factors are present. In order to directly view the outside of the reproductive organs so that endometriosis or adhesions can be visualized and treated, a laparoscopy is performed. This procedure is usually performed as a same-day procedure under general anesthesia in a hospital or outpatient surgical center. The abdomen is filled with carbon dioxide gas to create a hollow space. A small incision is made in the navel through which a narrow, lighted tube is inserted to allow visualization of the pelvic organs. Additional small incisions are made in the abdomen to allow insertion of surgical instruments. Many surgical procedures that could only be performed via a large incision can now be done laparoscopically, such as removal of endometriosis, ovarian cysts, and scar tissue. Recovery time depends on the amount of repair work that is performed and is generally a few days to a week.

Barriers to Implantation and Maintenance of Pregnancy

Infertility may be linked to problems in the development of the endometrium as well as the hormones that work to maintain pregnancy. These types of problems are often referred to as luteal phase defects. Several tests can be used to identify a luteal phase defect. First, a serum progesterone level may be performed by obtaining a blood sample approximately seven days after ovulation in order to determine if sufficient progesterone is produced to properly prepare the endometrium for implantation and pregnancy. Second, an endometrial biopsy may be performed so that endometrial tissue can be examined under the microscope for abnormalities in development. This testing is scheduled approximately one to three days prior to the next expected menstrual period. Before this test can be accomplished, a sensitive pregnancy test is performed to make sure that a much-wanted pregnancy is not disturbed. The biopsy is done by passing a thin tube through the cervical canal into the uterine cavity. A small amount of tissue is aspirated and the instrument is withdrawn. The woman may experience intense cramping during the procedure, which can be partly relieved by squirting local anesthetic into the uterine cavity prior to the test.

Third, a visual examination of the interior of the uterus may also be performed at the time of the laparoscopy. A hysteroscopy is done by inserting a lighted tube through the cervical canal into the uterine cavity. In this way, abnormalities of the uterine cavity that contribute to infertility, such as scar tissue, fibroid, or polyps, can be detected and removed.

Infertility Treatment

One of the most difficult aspects of treatment from both the physician and couple perspectives is the uncertainty of outcome and the lack of control over the outcome. There is not necessarily a correlation between identifying a problem, "correcting" it with treatment, and a resulting pregnancy. In fact, it seems as if the occurrence of pregnancy is more dependent on whether the sun, the moon, and the stars are aligned properly. If the physician were able to look into a crystal ball and tell the partners that they would never have a biological child, they would likely deal with the loss and get on with their lives. Likewise, if their physician were able to guarantee them a baby after the most grueling treatment, they would most likely go through it gladly. However, for partners more interested in determining whether they will and how they will conceive, there is a tremendous degree of uncertainty. In most other aspects of their lives, success is almost always assured by trying hard enough. With infertility treatment the rules are different: "Success" is defined as resolving the issue of infertility either through pregnancy, adoption, alternative parenting, or by making the decision to no longer actively pursue parenthood. The couple attains control when they carefully budget their emotional, financial, and social resources and when they determine how much time they will devote to infertility treatment.

With infertility treatment, knowing when to stop or move on is as difficult for the couple as it is for a gambler. All too often, a couple can become like a gambler who continues to put his coins into the slot machine, thinking that the next one will surely be the jackpot! To further the analogy, it is desirable in both examples to avoid emotional as well as financial bankruptcy. Both therapists and infertility care providers can provide the support necessary in order to prevent compulsive treatment. However, it is also important for the couple experiencing infertility to understand that the chances of conceiving are much better than winning in the casino and that Mother Nature weighs the odds in favor of conception. Infertility treatments are designed to give these processes a little push in the right direction.

Just as therapists have different styles and philosophies regarding psychotherapy, physicians who deal with infertility have different approaches to diagnosis and treatment. A competent provider tends to shape the treatment to the needs of the patient, rather than vice versa. Although there are many complicated medical options, dealing with infertility may not necessarily involve pushing the couple through each option, but rather helping the partners identify and choose from among them. It is well within the partners' rights to obtain certain information from their physician, such as the perceived cause of infertility, reasons for particular treatment options, an overview of the entire treatment plan, and a discussion about at what point they will be referred to a specialist. An important aspect of treatment, which helps them take an active role in their treatment and feel a sense of control, is the use of literature regarding infertility diagnosis and treatment, available to the physician for distribution to patients without cost.

Today, cost plays an important role when deciding which treatment option to pursue. Health insurance plans vary greatly in the amount and type of infertility treatments that will be covered. Many couples have no infertility coverage, placing the burden of the high costs of infertility treatments on credit cards, second mortgages, and prospective grandparents. As a result, infertility choices are frequently dictated by financial considerations rather than by medical efficacy of the treatments rendered. Decisions regarding treatment are also influenced by such factors as time commitment, age of the woman, convenience, and the many ethical issues surrounding infertility treatments. To some infertile couples, cost may be less relevant when weighing the increased time, frustration, and grief that may occur if the less successful procedures mean more failed cycles. Moreover, many couples are more interested in treatment that will achieve pregnancy within a reasonable time frame.

There are two different treatment philosophies that are utilized by physicians who treat infertility: (1) find out what's wrong and fix it or (2) nonspecifically enhance fertility by increasing the chances that the sperm and egg will get together. These two philosophies are not mutually exclusive but indicate the strain that can affect the couple's emotional, physical, and financial reserves. A physician who feels he or she must run the full gamut of testing may wear out the couple before they even get a chance at treatment. Likewise, treatment may be administered indefinitely without regard for the rule of diminishing returns: After three to four cycles of any treatment, chances for success diminish. This implies that if the treatment adequately addresses the infertility problem(s), pregnancy will occur promptly, whereas inappropriate treatment is not made more effective by continuing to pursue it. Therefore, if conception has not occurred after three to four cycles of a specific treatment, it is time to reevaluate the situation and plan the next step.

In recent years, there have been many advances in the treatment of infertility. For some infertility problems related to hormonal abnormalities, such as high prolactin levels, over- or underproduction of thyroid hormone, or polycystic ovarian syndrome (too much androgen produced by the ovaries or adrenal glands), normal hormonal levels can be restored with specific medication. In the case of high prolactin levels, bromocryptine is quite effective at normalizing serum levels but is unfortunately associated with orthostatic hypotension, nausea, and dizziness. High adrenal androgen levels can be normalized with small doses of dexamethasone, a synthetic steroid. If a thyroid problem is identified, thyroid hormone replacement can be provided.

The most common fertility medication used is clomiphene citrate, which is used to induce ovulation in women who do not ovulate on their own or enhances the ovulation of women who do ovulate. Clomiphene citrate enhances the release of FSH and LH from the pituitary, which in turn initiate follicular development and ovulation. Approximately 75 percent of anovulatory women will ovulate with clomiphene citrate and 35 percent will conceive. Clomiphene citrate is also used to empirically treat infertility when spontaneous ovulation is already occurring. Although this is a common use, it is controversial because of the relatively low pregnancy rates achieved and the long periods of time of treatment. In addition to its fertility-enhancing effects, clomiphene also has some antifertility actions that explain the relatively low conception rates with this drug. It can turn the cervical mucus into a barrier and also cause defects in the development of the endometrium. Therefore, clomiphene citrate should not be continued for more than three to four cycles before determining if these conditions exist or making a referral to an infertility specialist.

If diagnostic investigations find sperm problems, many treatment options are available. For men who have no sperm because of a mechanical blockage, congenital absence of sperm, or prior vasectomy, donor insemination is an option. Donors are carefully selected for their altruism, lack of high-risk sexual behavior, and good semen quality. The husbands are matched with a sperm donor on the basis of eye color, hair color, body build, and blood type. Semen samples from the donor are frozen in liquid nitrogen and thawed prior to use. The woman is inseminated with the donor's sperm at the time of ovulation with about a 20 percent chance of conceiving with each cycle. If conception has not occurred within four to six cycles, other causes of infertility should be sought in the woman.

Many couples come to a fertility specialist requesting donor insemination because they are aware of and accept the diagnosis of male infertility. Other couples may discover unexpectedly the presence of male sterility during the course of the infertility evaluation. Such a finding requires a considerable adjustment by both partners but generally affects the man more profoundly. In order to make sure that both partners are emotionally ready for donor insemination, many infertility specialists require that both partners be interviewed by a therapist prior to donor insemination, regardless of their situation. The interview also allows for discussion of other issues, such as attitudes about informing family and friends about the source of the sperm, whether and how to tell the child of his origin, and any other emotional issues.

The ideal approach to sperm abnormalities is to correct the problem. Some men have varicose veins of the testicles (varicocele) which are thought to increase the temperature of the testicles and adversely affect the quality of the sperm. If found, the varicoceles can be surgically treated and often the quality of the sperm improves sufficiently that a pregnancy results. Clomiphene citrate, which is comonly used in women to increase egg production, is sometimes used in the male to increase sperm counts.

Some men have low sperm counts but are potentially fertile if more sperm could reach the fallopian tubes. A laboratory procedure, known as intrauterine insemination (IUI), takes all the sperm in an ejaculated specimen, washes out the semen, and concentrates all the sperm in a very small volume of fluid. This fluid is then injected into the uterine cavity of the woman at the time of ovulation. In addition to overcoming some of the subfertility associated with low sperm counts, IUI is also used in cases of cervical mucus problems and antisperm antibodies and for nonspecifically enhancing fertility.

The combination of superovulation (stimulation of the ovary to produce multiple eggs) with IUI is a nonspecific method of enhancing fertility in couples with a variety of infertility problems, including anovulation, cervical mucus abnormalities, endometriosis, unexplained infertility, and advanced age. The only requirements for this treatment are that the fallopian tubes be open and that an adequate sperm count be present. While clomiphene citrate is often used to stimulate the ovary, the pregnancy rates per cycle are substantially better with human menopausal gonadotropins (hMG) (8 to 10 percent versus 12 to 30 percent). Treatment with hMG is rather expensive and requires daily injections as well as intensive ultrasound and serum hormone monitoring over a period of 10 to 12 days. Ovulation is triggered by an injection of human chorionic gonadotropin (hCG) when the eggs are determined to be of appropriate size. IUI is performed 36 to 42 hours after hCG as the eggs are released from the ovary. Superovulation with IUI is a standard infertility treatment with a high degree of success. However, the risks of multiple pregnancy (greater than twins) and ovarian hyperstimulation, which can be life threatening, make this treatment unattractive to some couples.

The surgical management of specific infertility problems has undergone considerable evolution over the past 25 years. Thus, there are a wide variety of approaches and the infertile couple should be encouraged to seek a second opinion if they are unsure of the approach that has been offered to them. Surgery to open blocked fallopian tubes, remove scar tissue, and remove endometriosis can be performed either by laparotomy or via laparoscopy. The former involves an abdominal incision, long recuperation, and the risk of formation of additional scar tissue. The latter is often referred to as "band-aid" surgery since the small incisions that are used can be covered with small dressings. Moreover, recovery is generally much faster and the risk of adhesion formation is less. However, laparoscopic surgery requires a level of surgical skill and experience that not every gynecologist possesses.

Advanced reproductive technologies (ART) offer hope for many couples, particularly those who have failed to conceive with other treatments. However, the knowledge that ART often represents treatment for "end-stage" infertility or is regarded as the "end of the line" adds considerable pressure to achieve success. ART treatment is also stressful because of the amount of medical intervention required to monitor response to treatment and the cost. In vitro fertilization (IVF) was the first of these new reproductive technologies that offered women with blocked tubes a chance to become pregnant. Additional "alphabet" techniques (GIFT, ZIFT) are variations of the IVF procedure and also provide hope for couples with unexplained infertility, severe male factor, and other forms of infertility unresponsive to more conservative treatment.

ART involves stimulating the ovary with large doses of hMG

(Pergonal, Humegon, Fertinex, or Metrodin) to stimulate the development of multiple eggs in the ovary. As the eggs develop, it is necessary to monitor blood estradiol levels and perform vaginal ultrasounds frequently; all of these require a significant time commitment. When the eggs are believed to be ripe by these determinations, the woman is given an injection of hCG, which causes final maturation of the eggs. Transvaginal retrieval of the eggs must be accomplished prior to release of the eggs, which occurs 36 to 42 hours after hCG. After the eggs are harvested, the husband must produce a semen sample so that the sperm and eggs can be incubated together. A day later the couple finds out if fertilization has occurred. Transfer of the embryo(s) occurs 24 hours later by guiding a thin tube containing the embryos into the uterine cavity.

IVF technology is rapidly expanding to provide couples additional options. For men with very low or abnormal sperm counts, a laboratory procedure, known as intracytoplasmic sperm injection (ICSI), is available in which an individual sperm is inserted into an egg. Novel methods of semen collection from men who produce no sperm are also being developed. To improve implantation, some labs are now using assisted hatching that enhances the ability of the embryo to break through the zona pelucida, the outer shell of the egg.

As much as ART has become a precise science, it also remains very much an art and subject to the same astrological influences as other types of infertility treatment. Success of ART is dependent on the number and quality of eggs, fertilization, compulsive attention to detail in the lab, and many other factors that cannot be identified and therefore are uncontrollable. Individual women's responses to these treatments may vary and disappointments are possible at any point along this sequence of events. For example, the woman may not develop any eggs, there may be premature release of the eggs from the ovary, no eggs may be obtained from the ovary, the semen sample may be inadequate, stage fright may prevent the husband from producing his contribution, fertilization may not occur, and they may get a negative pregnancy test. These are viewed as potential losses and contribute to increased anxiety even before a cycle is initiated. For every 100 couples who go through one cycle of IVF, approximately 25 to 30 will hit the jackpot and conceive. The remainder of the couples has to make the difficult decision of trying again or moving on.

For women who do not produce eggs because of age or ovarian failure, or for women who fail IVF due to age or high FSH levels, egg donation provides an encouraging alternative. A friend, family member, or anonymous donor undergoes stimulation of her ovaries as described above. The eggs are retrieved and fertilized with the sperm from the prospective father. The embryos are transferred to the wife, who has been appropriately prepared with hormones. While this can be an expensive procedure, which sometimes involves a long wait for a donor (up to a year or more), it provides the opportunity to experience pregnancy and childbirth firsthand.

Ethics of Treatment

The scientific advances that have created the technology to help so many couples achieve their goal of a family have also created ethical issues that lead to questions such as, "Just because we can, should we?" Couples who barely have a functional understanding of normal reproductive processes may have a difficult time understanding the complexities of the reproductive technology as well as the ethical issues. Out of their desire for a child, they may ask for treatments that are within our abilities technologically, but may raise significant ethical issues on the part of the physician and staff. These couples may question why they should be "denied" a chance at pregnancy because of ethical concerns that do not bother them. Such issues are discussed in detail in chapter 8.

For example, consider the case of a couple seeking identified sperm donation using the prospective paternal grandfather's sperm. While all participants want to keep the genetic lineage within the family and avoid the remote chance of acquiring a sexually transmitted disease, they also raise issues of potential use of an unequal power base, paternal pressure, and even incest. The physician who is uncomfortable offering this specific treatment can explain his or her reasons to the couple, offer them anonymous sperm donation, or same-generation identified sperm donation, or refer the couple to another physician who may be willing to offer the type of treatment which they desire.

Resolution of Infertility

The most desired type of resolution of infertility is conception and pregnancy. For the partners who have reached their limits emotionally, financially, or temporally, the road to parenthood may not be over. However, the transition from actively pursuing treatment to accepting failure of that particular route will involve considerable emotional turmoil. When should couples stop treatment? How much is enough? What if they tried just one more time? What if they tried treatment with another physician? The therapist and the infertility physician can do much to support the couple struggling with these questions. Treatments should be offered for a limited number of cycles and couples should be encouraged to discuss their emotional and financial limitations so that they can budget their resources effectively. Discussions of alternative plans for parenthood should begin before the partners have reached their limit. Couples who stop infertility treatments before they have exhausted all of the possible steps should not be made to feel that they are failures. Rather they should be encouraged to explore other parenting options.

Once a couple accepts the fact that infertility treatments will not yield biological parenthood, the partners can more readily consider the alternatives of adoption, other alternative parenting, such as being a good aunt and uncle, or child-free living.

2
THE COUPLE'S DEVELOPMENTAL CYCLE

WHEN JASON AND LISA ARRIVED IN my office for their first therapy session, they had been separated for two months. They had been married for ten years, five of which had been spent undergoing grueling and painful infertility procedures. Prior to their struggles with infertility they had negotiated many of the hurdles young couples encounter. They had passed through the various stages of forming a relationship, which helped define the character of their marriage. Jason and Lisa had reorganized their individual identities and begun to work as a unit, a system of integrated parts. But they were stymied by the disappointments and stresses of the infertility experience. When they confronted infertility they realized their bodies were not working as well-integrated parts. As a result of all of the stress and discouragement, they realized their marriage was not functioning as a well-integrated, effective system either.

As Todd (1986) explains, the behavior of the couple system is influenced by the personalities of each of the partners as well as such factors as the impact of children, the couple's respective families of origin, friends, and work systems. The partners have to continually work to define their boundaries and their interaction with all of these systems, a complex process that is further complicated by the fact that "the dyad is considered to be a goal-oriented system that attempts to satisfy the competing needs of the individual partners, the couple as an entity, and those of the environment" (Todd, p. 72). All couples, whether heterosexual, gay, lesbian, married, or unmarried, must struggle to negotiate and define these complex interactions. The desire to accommodate all of these demands pushes the partners to try to make some sense out of their worlds and their needs, but also results in added stress on their relationship.

Like most young couples, Jason and Lisa had looked to their relationship as a source of support and sustenance. Each believed the other was the one who would always understand and love them no matter what. Their marriage would be the solution to their problems. They would never be lonely again. They would always have someone to support them. As Carter and McGoldrick (1989) emphasize, a wedding, the union of two individuals, represents more than a rite of passage; the wedding is often seen by the couple and their families as a terminating process. Parents feel their child is "grown-up and settled" at last. The wedding symbolizes the beginning of an intricate process of changing family status. Jason and Lisa could not have predicted how challenging the various aspects of marriage would be.

Jason and Lisa met on a balmy summer night at a party hosted by Lisa's friend Julie. Jason was immediately drawn to Lisa. He was attracted to her physically, and he was also quite taken by her laughter and her "dancing eyes," as he explained. He thought her eyes indicated a playfulness and enthusiasm, which appealed to him. Lisa, on the other hand, was not immediately attracted to Jason. She thought he was arrogant and too serious. However, his intense pursuit finally paid off when she decided to date him. Much to her surprise she found his seriousness admirable. She was quite impressed with his success, and she found that behind his arrogance was really a gentle, almost shy, person—a complement to her strong personality. She quickly responded to his manner and his wry humor. Although she had been reluctant to become involved in a relationship at that point in her life, she found herself rapidly "falling for" Jason.

All her life Lisa had imagined her Prince Charming: someone as handsome and successful as Jason. Being with him made her feel strong. She knew she was competent and successful, but Jason made her feel even more valuable, more whole. She admired and loved his intensity. He was more powerful than her dad. He liked his work and was committed to it, so he wouldn't need her to be there with him all the time, and he would understand her independence.

Jason thought Lisa was the perfect partner. She was independent and had her own identity, yet she would be a charming "corporate wife," pretty and bubbly. She was warm and loving, unlike his critical, demanding mom. He could relax and be himself with her and she loved it. She thought he was funny and clever and she made him feel powerful and sexy.

And so the relationship continued to develop. Each individual became part of the pair. They became a couple and developed a "we" language with one another and with their friends. Jason and Lisa experienced many tumultuous ups and downs as they struggled with their relationship issues and their individual needs; they were two distinct personalities attempting to merge into a viable couple. Although they knew they wanted to marry and spend their lives together, they could not anticipate the enormity of what they were about to encounter: the evolution of their marital system with a life of its own.

Relationships need to accommodate both the individuals' needs and the couple's growth needs. Even though all marriages have distinguishing aspects and are essentially unique, all lasting relationships go through some of the same sequential phases and require the completion of common relationship tasks. According to Nichols (1988), the development of a marriage is similar to individual and family development, in that the marital life cycle also follows predictable stages. At each stage there are specific tasks to be mastered if the relationship is to move from its inception through the death of one of the partners without experiencing separation or divorce.

As Jason and Lisa continued the struggle to define their couple system, they passed through some of the normal phases of couple development. As Bader and Pearson (1988) explain, these maturational milestones create a deeper bonding in the relationship and the ability to increase relationship skills. The development of the relationship involves a progression through successive stages. Each stage represents a transformation of an earlier stage into a more complex form. The growth process is thus one of transformation, for both the couple and the individuals within the system. Although couple and family growth processes are not linear, the processes exist in a linear dimension of time (Carter & McGoldrick, 1989). However, since the stages are successive, failure to negotiate a particular phase becomes a source of conflict and divisiveness in the relationship, which severely disrupts the couple's growth and development.

The complexity of the marital relationship requires that the spouses learn to negotiate together issues they have previously defined individually or defined within the context of their families of origin (Carter & McGoldrick, 1989). The issues, ranging from simply where, when, and how to sleep, eat, work, or relax, to the more involved issues around fighting, their sexual relationship, and interactions with extended families, all become challenges to their relationship. The couple cannot resolve these issues and simply move forward because the relationship is not linear. As Dym and Glenn (1993) explain, once the spouses resolve an issue, they do not remain at the resolution point forever. They continue to adjust, since the character of their couple system is constantly evolving.

Stages in the Couple's Development

Jason could clearly describe his initial attraction to Lisa and articulate his present unhappiness with her: "She used to laugh so much and be so lighthearted, but now she is withdrawn and sullen so much of the time." Both could recall the early phase of their relationship, the romance and enchantment. Lisa explained how she often felt "madly in love with Jason." Such feelings are clearly representative of the first of three stages of couple relationships described by Dym and Glenn (1993).

During the initial stage, expansion and promise, the spouses focus on their desire to connect, to transcend the isolation, become more vulnerable, and join with each other. Feelings of infatuation and romance are an important aspect of this stage. The second stage, contraction and betrayal, involves struggles with disillusionment. Spouses experience more pessimism as the realities of everyday life impact the relationship and they sometimes see their partner falter. As the infatuation begins to fade, they become more comfortable going in separate directions and more distant or even cynical. However, because of their commitment to one another, they struggle past the pessimism to arrive at the third stage, resolution. The struggle to reach a compromise creates calm and some stability, which takes them back to some of the romance and connectedness of their early relationship. However, the peace experienced during resolution is interrupted when another life circumstance, such as the birth of a child or the loss of a parent, impacts the couple. The stages then recycle, with some of the same dynamics occurring.

Heiman, Epps, and Ellis (1995) propose three interactional patterns that influence a couple's sense of togetherness or separateness. Although they are not necessarily sequential, the interactions impact how the couple defines their relationship at different times. The first involves the struggle with territoriality—the rights of ownership of physical or psychological space, such as one's body or household territory. The second interactional pattern relates to issues of attachment, or how the couple deals with interactions around intimacy, affection, and fluctuations in intensity between them. The third pattern is ranking order, or how the couple struggles with issues of status, dominance, and power.

Nichols (1988) defines the couple's stages more broadly. Although he might agree that couples struggle with the principles of interaction described by Heiman and colleagues and need to accomplish numerous tasks during the various stages, he describes the stages in a life cycle developmental context. Nichols begins with what he labels the mating and marriage stage. This stage involves establishing the marital boundary by defining a couple identity. An additional and important task of this stage requires separating from one's family of origin. This stage is similar to Dym and Glenn's (1993) expansion stage, because the focus is on the establishment of the couple identity and beginning the processes of defining themselves as separate from their families of origin.

The second stage of the marriage begins with the decision to have a child. Nichols (1988) labels *this* the expansion stage. The spouses work to define their couple identity and simultaneously struggle with the issue of parenthood, since it is crucial to the adult developmental task of generativity (Erikson, 1950). They begin to fulfill their parental roles as a couple, necessitating that the boundaries of the marriage and the new family be clearly delineated. The couple struggles with becoming a nuclear family, with new roles and new rules. As the spouses make room for a new family member and define their nuclear family, there is a reorganization of power and a reworking of the power relationship with their parents (Nichols, 1988). Struggling through such change forces the partners to further refine their marriage. Clarification of the marital relationship is crucial during this stage, since the task of developing together is more challenging at this point than at any other in the marriage. The internal and external responsibilities loom large. As each partner struggles with parenting, individual development, and career aspirations, they may discover they have developed along different paths at different rates. They may discover they have little left in common other than their offspring. They need to frequently rework their relationship and find new ways to define it and to continue to find meaning within the marital dyad.

Contraction, the third stage of the marital life cycle, involves the challenges of the separation and individuation of the children. The challenge for the couple is to keep in touch with the growth of each family member, and to understand and respect their emotional and intellectual growth. Subsequently, with the encroaching arrival of the empty nest, the spouses struggle to regenerate the marital relationship as a dyad, to again begin to regard one another as the most important person in their world.

During the postparental years, the fourth stage according to Nichols (1988), individuals focus on the attempt to find meaning and satisfaction in the context of decreasing abilities. Among the more painful tasks of this stage are learning to deal with both realized and anticipated losses. The partners have adapted to the separation from their children and the loss related to this process. Now they have to struggle with the potential loss of one another as well as anticipate the more imminent loss of their own parents.

The above three classifications of couple's stages are more complementary than mutually exclusive. Each contributes to an understanding of the dynamic ebb and flow of a couple's ongoing struggles. Dym and Glenn's stages are more descriptive of relationship processes than developmental stages, even though they are cyclical. Heiman and colleagues discuss stages and tasks, but they are less extensive than the stages Nichols proposes. It is understandable that when two individuals marry, their individual maturation processes combine to create a complex sequence of developmental stages that parallel the stages of individual growth and development. Since Nichols' model integrates many of these parallel developmental tasks, it is a more thorough explanation of two individuals struggling through their own developmental sequences within the couple dyad.

Table 2.1 summarizes our discussion of a couple's developmental cycle. So, even as the marital life cycle comes to a close, new relationships evolve and ultimately generate new life. And so the cycle of life continues—that is, unless the couple encounters a glitch, such as the crisis of infertility.

Romantic Notions and Expectations

Most young people mature with the notion that they will one day have a meaningful long-term relationship and will then create their own families. Jason thought Lisa was the perfect "girl of my dreams." She would be an ideal partner and mother for his children. Jason also fulfilled Lisa's picture of her Prince Charming; she imagined a fulfilling life with him and thought about what a great father he would be.

However, some individuals expect too much from a partner. They may fuse with the other in an attempt to gain strength or resolve a feeling of loneliness. They look to the other for a sense of wholeness. Sometimes they are running away from their families of origin or seeking the family they never had (Carter & McGoldrick, 1989). Sometimes the anticipation of parenthood is an attempt to avoid—or complete—unfinished developmental tasks (Gutman, 1985).

Jason and Lisa were not seeking to escape their families of origin, but rather to improve upon them. Even so, they experienced disillusionment as they learned the other was not the magic wizard who could wave the wand and make life perfect. "I thought Jason was so perfect that he would make our life perfect," explained Lisa one afternoon. "Then it was such a long hard fall when I realized that even he couldn't right all the wrongs; even Jason

TABLE 2.1. THE COUPLE'S DEVELOPMENTAL CYCLE

STUDY	STAGE	TASKS/ISSUES
Dym & Glenn (1993)	Expansion and promise	Connect; become vulnerable
	Contraction and betrayal	Struggle with disillusionment; face the realities of partner
	Resolution	Arrive at a comfortable balance of closeness/distance
Heiman, Epps, & Ellis (1995)	Defining territoriality	Rights of ownership
	Issues of attachment	Intimacy, affection, intensity
	Ranking order	Status, dominance, power
Nichols (1988)	Mating and marriage	Establish marital boundary; separate from families of origin; establish communication, conflict management, and sexual relationship
	Expansion	Adjust to becoming a nuclear family; learn to fulfill parental roles as individual and couple; redefine relationships with family of origin
	Contraction	Rework expectations of couple relationship; let go of children; deal with empty nest
	Postparental	Find meaning and satisfaction in the context of declining abilities; realign relationships with all generations

couldn't change the course of things and make a baby happen." Jason chimed in somewhat defensively, "I began to harbor resentment toward Lisa because I could feel that she expected so much of me. I felt helpless, impotent I guess. It sure didn't make me feel sexy or romantically disposed toward Lisa." The challenges and disappointments of infertility were quickly eroding their fairy tale and the larger-than-life romantic notions that had permeated their early relationship.

The infertility experience is exacerbated by the fact that in most other aspects of their functioning these individuals have been very successful. Particularly if they have purposely delayed childbearing, they are usually established and respected in their career endeavors. At this juncture then, when they confront the infertility, they may believe they are failing to develop and mature normally. They perceive their childless condition as a personal failure rather than a cruel twist of nature. This was the case with Paul and Sandy, both physicians in their late thirties, who were shocked when confronted with their infertility.

Paul and Sandy had met in medical school, but it was not an immediate infatuation. "We were just good friends at first," explained Paul. "We studied together with the same group of friends and found we could really talk. We were always so comfortable together." Sandy smiled and continued their story, "We even began to spend holidays at one another's parents' because we all felt like one big happy family. For a long time we were more like cousins than dating partners. And then one day something just clicked, really at the same time for both of us, and the relationship took a romantic turn."

They married and decided to postpone having children in order to travel, build their house, and just have some fun. Paul, a sensitive and shy man, was able to articulate their sense of failure, "We had so much to do and were having a good time, so we decided to postpone our decision about children." Sandy added, "We spent so many years getting through medical school that we just wanted to play together without having to account to a needy infant. Eight years later, when we finally decided it was time to have a baby, I didn't anticipate that I wouldn't be able to get pregnant. I didn't think I was defective."

Even though Sandy considered herself successful and quite competent in her career, her infertility created much self-doubt and deprecation. She blamed herself and her body for her inability to succeed at such an important life goal. What she had not appreciated until later in their therapy was the meaning she and Paul attributed to having a child. They had to look carefully at their motives for having, or not having, a child. They had to examine how infertility might affect their decision about parenthood.

Paul and Sandy realized that part of their quandary related to the fact that they have many choices their parents did not have. The combination of recent medical advances and social and economic changes in the culture have led couples like Paul and Sandy to feel an increased desire to control and manage their fertility (Gutman, 1985). Ironically, they had focused most of their time on controlling their fertility rather than on creating their own nuclear family.

However, they were also influenced by their relationships with their own families of origin. Even though they had enjoyed spending time with each other's families during their early friendship and dating years, they both were insightful about their unresolved difficulties with their families and were able to discuss these issues together. "Paul was always a good friend," Sandy explained. "I could tell him how my mom drove me crazy—how overprotective she was, and how she was always offering an opinion, always sticking her nose into my business. And I know that sometimes I looked too much for her approval or opinion." Sandy's unresolved fusion with her parents influenced her deferred childbearing. Because she was still overly tied to her parents, she feared becoming overwhelmed by the needs of a totally dependent infant.

"We had some problems, too, because of this strong attachment Sandy had with her parents," Paul continued. "Not only did that bond create turmoil for Sandy, because she often felt tremendous pressure to be the 'good daughter,' but it also created a tension between us, because she felt so much pressure to do her parents' bidding. Sometimes I felt she was more loyal to them than to me; yet, other times I felt smothered by her constant soliciting of what I felt, how I felt, or what I might advise her to do." Sandy's unresolved dependency, or fusion, issues resulted in an ambivalence related to some level of recognition that because of the fusion in the marriage, the couple's pseudointimacy would be threatened by the injection of an infant into the system (Gutman, 1985).

Individuals who have successfully passed through each developmental stage feel a desire to do things together (Bader & Pearson, 1988). They are comfortable with the intimacy in their dyad and in fact enjoy it. Therefore, the anticipation of a child reinforces their desire for togetherness instead of threatening them. Whereas in the earlier stages of the marriage one spouse may have become upset when the other desired space, at this more differentiated stage separateness in fact strengthens the marital bond. Paradoxically, the couple can focus on the joint venture of creating a family as a result of their separateness.

Loss, Betrayal, and Disillusionment

A couple's progression through the appropriate stages of development can stall when the couple is confronted with infertility. Since most men and women reach adulthood with the assumption that they will eventually become parents, couples experience a strong sense of betrayal and confusion when they face infertility. "Being a mother or father is a primary source of self-identity. The two individuals involved construct identities about who they are and where and how they fit into the world and construct social definitions consonant with the social definition of marriage and family" (Atwood & Dobkin, 1992, p. 393). Therefore, as parenthood continues to elude these individuals, they do not know where they stand in terms of defining themselves as individuals or as a couple.

When Jason and Lisa confronted the infertility crisis, they realized no one could rescue them from this demon. They had to acknowledge what they considered a failure to achieve one of life's milestones. Young adults moving toward the stage of generativity feel that having children is "the first, and for many, the prime generative encounter" (Erikson, 1964, p. 130). So couples who encounter infertility problems struggle with both individual and marital life cycle developmental crises. The crises result not wholly from the medical aspects of the problem, but also from the sudden disruption in expectations (Butler & Koraleski, 1990). All they had planned and taken for granted has now been threatened.

So these individuals feel at odds with society, betrayed by nature, their bodies, and one another. Also, because reproduction represents the survival and continuity of the family and the species, the couple has to struggle with the symbolic aspects that such a loss portends. The spouses are forced to examine the meaning they ascribed to their progeny. They are now forced to question their commitment to having children within the context of the rising emotional and financial costs of infertility. They did not choose to be different. They became accustomed to having many options. They realized their ability to make crucial life decisions far exceeded that of any generation before them. Therefore, it was incomprehensible that such a crucial decision could be stolen from them.

Nichols (1988) believes that couples without children, whether they have chosen to be child-free, that is, to deliberately focus on other rewarding life options, or to remain sadly childless, go through the same developmental stages as those who produce and rear children, excepting the stages directly related to parenting. However, many couples struggling with infertility would disagree. Paul and Sandy can readily express how the issues surrounding the infertility negatively affected their marriage, how the medical investigations highlighted problems with their sexual functioning, communication, and therefore their general marital satisfaction. They can also describe how their friends who did not experience infertility shifted more easily through the developmental stages.

The infertility crisis magnifies the disappointment and hurt that couples in a conventional developmental sequence experience. "Regardless of etiology, failure to produce a desired conception seems to create varied and intense reactions for couples" (Gutman, 1985, p. 137). Such partners are forced to intensely face one another in order to reevaluate their life purpose and deal with their deep disappointment. In this process they frequently turn on one another, even with the full realization that their partner hurts just as much and is just as helpless to resolve the crisis. They may feel even more defeated and powerless because they did not choose this life course.

"If we are not able to fulfill our dreams of creating our family," cried Sandy during one therapy session, "then I'll just feel like a weirdo, kind of bouncing along with life's tide. I have no meaning or purpose anymore. Here I always thought all I needed was my career and that my career would always be sort of a buffer for any life disappointments. But what a surprise!" Paul added, "I started to get angry with Sandy because I was being cheated out of something I'd always assumed would be part of my life. I felt betrayed. I felt our bodies betrayed us. I have always defined myself as a successful breadwinner for my family. I always assumed I would have that role for my family—but now maybe I won't even have that family. I don't know how to act anymore with my family or friends." Paul no longer had the script originally given to him by his family and his culture that told him both how to behave and how to achieve these goals (Atwood & Dobkin, 1992).

Spouses faced with infertility experience changes in their world view about what is fair, about goals, self-worth; feelings of attractiveness and prowess are also challenged. The childless condition continues to confront them like an enormous brick wall they cannot get through, around, or over. Feelings of loss and betrayal surround them. There are multiple losses: loss of children, genetic continuity, pregnancy, control, and loss of an important life goal (Valentine, 1986). They have lost a sense of balance with all generations: their own, their parents, and their imagined children's. "In any case, infertility is a medical, psychological, and social experience requiring a redefinition by the couple of their identities as individuals and as partners" (McDaniel, Hepworth, & Doherty, 1992, p. 106).

The experience of infertility is all-consuming because it involves both an individual process and a couple process (Cooper & Glazer, 1994). The ways in which the couple assumed they would balance the roles of parent, spouse, or breadwinner require renegotiation. Issues of power and money and perhaps even the marital duties all have to be reexamined. Even beyond these necessary changes with the marital dynamics, the couple has to reexamine family of origin expectations as well as the complicated issues surrounding how and when to interact with extended family members.

It is not only the young couple but also the families of origin who feel the threatened loss of the family's future. Infertility is an intergenerational crisis. Often the parents of the infertile couple wonder if somehow they caused this "defect." They search their memories trying to remember childhood illnesses or other physical problems this son or daughter experienced. They feel guilty even if there is no possible correlation between childhood experiences and the couple's current infertility condition.

Further, the potential lack of future generations doesn't allow for mending or correcting generational problems. The couple may have believed they could have done better with their children, thus repairing many of their dysfunctional family dynamics. They may also have wished that their child or children could help improve or repair their relationship with their parents. Thus they experience further loss. Relationships with siblings who have children or are pregnant can become strained or even cut off, which can further threaten the survival of the family and certainly increase everyone's sense of loss.

Deviation from the Cultural Narrative

Our culture asks so much of couple relationships that disappointment is inevitable. Most individuals initially perceive their relationship as a cure-all for loneliness. They expect their partner to be an everlasting friend, lover, and confidant, the one who will always be "my everything." Eventually such demands become a burden for the couple system. The system cannot maintain the romance and passion in light of all of life's trials. "We all begin with a growing sense of elation and expansion, a sense of promise that seems bigger than life. And sooner or later, we all stumble. We start arguing, see our life together as less than it originally seemed, and enter a time of contraction" (Dym & Glenn, 1993, p. 11).

Couples experiencing the infertility crisis stumble harder and sometimes sooner than other couples. Their sense of expansiveness as a couple and a family is prematurely halted. They are challenged by the shock of what is not occurring in their lives. More than other couples, infertile couples find "the expansive promise of new beginnings often comes to seem like a youthful illusion, at best—a cruel hoax, at worst" (Dym & Glenn, 1993, p. xiv). What they had taken for granted, their hopes and dreams about family, instead become painful lessons of life's course.

A further source of pain for these couples relates to the prescribed composite that dictates the right and wrong ways to function in our society. The "cultural narrative," as Dym and Glenn (1993) label it, tells individuals how and when they should or shouldn't live together, whether and when they should marry, and the preferred rites and routines they should follow. The prescriptives are specific and unyielding. As a result, those who do not follow the path struggle with feeling defective and punished. "They are punished internally, through discomfort and shame; and externally by the representatives of society—employers, parents, the in-crowd, etc.," who regard them with disdain and disapproval (Dym & Glenn, p. 40).

The irony, however, is that couples experiencing infertility are punished not only by the infertility itself but also by society because they do not conform to conventional developmental sequences. They are regarded as aberrant by family, friends, and the larger culture. Further, since parenting is often a basic component of the marriage, the marriage may be threatened when the parenting function is threatened. And because "negative events for which one is potentially responsible pose the greatest threat to emotional well-being" (McEwan, Costello, & Taylor, 1987, p. 113), the partners worry that they may have deprived the other of a more "normal" life experience. Each suffers with their own loss and the fear that perhaps they will be blamed.

"I wanted so much to feel normal, to fit in," Lisa cried during one session, "I blamed Jason and blamed myself. We didn't ask for this. We didn't freely make the decision to not have a child. So why are we regarded like such pariahs?" Lisa could not make sense of the coercive forces the cultural narrative creates. She only knew she had experienced their power and thus her own sense of powerlessness. "I don't understand why I can't get beyond this," she sighed. "I've always been accepted and popular. Now I feel like I don't belong. People don't know what to say to me or even how to ask how I am." Her entire context had become contaminated by this twist of nature.

Lisa also began to realize the importance of redefining her and Jason's goals, as well as their relationship, if the marriage were to survive. "Deviation from the cultural narrative may thus precipitate developmental shifts in the couple and developmental shifts may help the couple reinterpret their fit with the cultural narrative" (Dym & Glenn, 1993, p. 39).

Jason and Lisa began to see how they had become more separate, blamed one another, and turned inward in response to feeling awkward and aberrant. They learned how they had turned on each other when they didn't understand their pain. And they learned the importance of redefining themselves and their relationship in order to transcend the rigid societal prescriptives. "I felt so misunderstood by Lisa, our friends, and our families," Jason said toward the end of their therapy. "I couldn't understand why our friends regarded us as outcasts or why our families sometimes seemed irritated or impatient with us. Now I can see they probably thought we were selfish and indulgent. I felt we had failed them, but didn't understand why or how. I get it now. I began to get this perspective, to realize how we begin our lives with such hope and optimism. Then, as we master more of our world, both physically and intellectually, we think we can do it all. You know, the invincible years of adolescence and early adulthood. And then I found my Princess Charming, so I thought I was even more powerful. And then, boom, this huge meteor called infertility comes out of nowhere and crashes on us. So we grow up. We realize that life isn't a bowl of cherries, like our parents tried to tell us. I don't feel angry or weird anymore, but I sure do long for that youthful innocence of our early marriage."

3

THE EMOTIONAL STAGES OF
THE INFERTILITY CRISIS

INFERTILITY IS ONE OF THE MOST difficult stressors a couple can face. The diagnostic and treatment procedures are psychologically and physically overwhelming. The couple endures countless emotional and physical trials in order to accommodate the demanding medical procedures. The infertility process begins to permeate all aspects of the spouses' lives. They have to contend with it during their workday, through appointments and telephone exchanges, and in the evening, when discussing test results and future plans. The shock and disbelief they feel about the possibility of not having the family they fantasized create intense emotional reactions for each individual as well as the marital system. As they continue through treatment, they become more acutely aware of each particular day of the wife's cycle and her body's nuances. They experience a chronic monthly hope-loss cycle. The devastation worsens each month (McDaniel, Hepworth, & Doherty, 1992) and their reserve for dealing with the pain diminishes. They are on a monthly emotional roller coaster, alternating between calm acceptance and highly intense emotional outbursts (Atwood & Dobkin, 1992).

The process intensifies as the spouses begin to realize that they may not be able to have a biological child. The spouses go through stages of mourning much like they would with terminal illness or the death of a loved one. They experience a deep sense of loss each month with the onset of menstruation (Atwood & Dobkin, 1992). The stages of mourning are similar to those described by Kübler-Ross (1969), such as denial, anger, and depression, but with certain differences in the dynamics, the progression, and the intensity (Cook, 1987; Eck Menning, 1980, 1984). For example, if the husband is terminally ill, the wife may be angry because of his anticipated abandonment. With infertilty, one partner may experience anger toward the impaired partner because he is depriving her of a dream. Additionally, in the case of infertility, the "illness" that they are grieving is rarely life threatening, but can be quite threatening to the marital system. Further, the illness may not serve to bring them—or their families—closer.

And so the couple begins an unanticipated and grueling journey through the stages associated with infertility. The spouses will experience an unfolding sequence of hope and devastation, of promise and disappointment, that will challenge them beyond anything they have experienced individually or in their marriage.

Effects of Infertility on the Marital System

Shock and Disbelief

Initially, the partners experience disbelief, surprise, or shock. They had always taken their fertility for granted. Carol and Bob were a dynamic pair, the envy of many of their friends. Both had very successful careers in management positions with different community hospitals. Both were close to their families of origin, and as they entered their mid-thirties, the issue of starting their own family became more prominent. Carol explained her reactions well: "We had built a stable foundation for a family. We had reached a good point in our careers, we had bought our dream house, and then we were ready for our family. We just couldn't believe it when we weren't pregnant within six months. Everything else had worked so well when we decided the time was right. I just kept making excuses. I was in shock."

Denial

The feeling of shock the couple experiences may evolve into denial. Partners may use many excuses to explain the monthly disappointment. "I never dreamed of infertility," Carol said. "I just attributed the nonpregnancy to stress or to the bad bout of flu I'd had. We even had some fights about not making love frequently enough." As with most failure or loss, Carol and Bob deny the severity of their situation until they find a way to make sense of it. They attempt to manage their lives as normally as possible, minimizing the disruption, when in fact the diagnostics and treatment regimens are severely disruptive and demanding. They deny the nagging fear that they may never realize their dream. Initially, denial can reduce the stress, but eventually they must learn more adaptive coping mechanisms so they do not put their physical or psychological welfare at risk (Callan & Hennessey, 1989). They must face the realities of their problem and prognosis.

Anxiety

As the partners continue to struggle with their disappointment, they begin to acknowledge their difficulty with fertility, their sense of helplessness with their problem, and their increasing anxiety. They are anxious about what this might mean for their relationship. Each fears being identified as "the problem." They worry whether they can survive together if they cannot realize this life dream. "I'm so worried that Carol will leave me if we can't get pregnant," Bob confessed one session. "I know how important family is for her, and I know how badly she's wanted kids. I especially worry if I'm the one with the problem—you know, if somehow I'm infertile or something, that she'll see me as inadequate or incomplete and won't love me anymore." If they have begun a diagnostic workup, they are anxious about the vulnerable parts of themselves, both physical and psychological, that are under examination. Their self-esteem is threatened as they are poked and prodded and questioned. They begin to question their completeness or defectiveness. Each partner becomes more concerned about his or her personal adequacy and about the outcomes of this prodding and questioning. Each feels increasingly anxious as the diagnostic tests become more complicated and intrusive. The couple becomes immersed in a medical-psychological vicious cycle, which further increases the partners' anxiety. Life revolves more and more around the diagnostics and the focus on pregnancy—or the lack thereof. The partners push themselves forward, hoping that the next procedure will be the wonderful solution. Or, with dashed hopes they struggle with the disappointment, feel more anxious, but again muster all the strength they have to enter the next round of medical interventions. And so the cycle continues.

Anger

It is not surprising that the couple begins to experience anger. Each partner feels cheated at not being able to easily achieve a life goal he or she had taken for granted. One may feel angry at the other or begin to resent the other. Although Carol bragged about their dream house and indicated in their early therapy sessions that they had concurred about their decision to be more settled before having children, in a later session she grabbed the opportunity to vent her anger: "I'm so angry with him I don't know whether I can forgive him. He always drags his feet on important decisions. I wanted to discuss having kids when we turned thirty. But old conservative Bob wanted to wait until we were more settled financially and stable in our careers. So we waited and now look where we are!"

A partner may also be angry and resentful about the other partner's impaired fertility; he or she may even openly admit thoughts of finding another partner. The impaired partner may offer to "let" the fertile one out of the marriage. The marital system becomes threatened, adding an additional component of potential loss. The individuals then become concerned about having to choose between their marriage and the child they desperately want. They struggle with a lose-lose situation: to lose this spouse or to possibly lose the desired biological child.

An angry, hurt spouse may look for someone on whom to blame the infertility. The partner is often the first target, although sometimes a parent is blamed because she didn't explain adequately about the potential dangers of an IUD or because she took DES when pregnant. A spouse may project anger at those who choose abortion or about reports of child abuse (Atwood & Dobkin,

1992). The couple may turn blame on the medical team or the medical community as a whole. Such collusion may serve to unite the spouses, but merely becomes another unconstructive way to deal with the anger and underlying pain.

Loss of Control

As they work their way through the medical maze, the partners experience a series of procedures that are often costly and painful and intrude into their private relationships (Berg & Wilson, 1991). The infertility evaluation itself adds stress as past sexual behaviors and reproductive histories are explored. The partners become wrapped up a whirl of appointments, decisions, and the monitoring of their bodies and sex lives. They experience an increased sense of loss of control. What used to be predictable in their lives is no longer. They find it difficult to plan. Can they take a vacation next month, or will that come at a critical time in their cycle? Carol and Bob were able to articulate how the sense of loss of control extended to their careers, making that part of their life feel out of control too. Bob had an important business trip he needed to plan, but was stymied about when to schedule it. "What if that's 'the crucial time' and I'm thousands of miles away? Maybe Carol could schedule a rendezvous part way!" he said sarcastically. Similarly, Carol expressed how her career had been on hold for over a year: "I kept ignoring discussions about a promotion even though I wanted more challenge because I thought I'd become pregnant at any time and then not want more challenge. Besides, I didn't want added stress and another adjustment in my life right now with all of the stress of the infertility workups."

Isolation and Alienation

The chronic nature of the psychological pain leads the couple to isolate themselves. The partners feel more alienated as their friends become pregnant; they have less in common with these friends, who are absorbed with creating their families. They believe their friends tire of hearing about their infertility ups and downs. They may feel embarrassed because they are different. This self-imposed isolation and alienation may reinforce feelings of being defective, which further isolate them. They want support, and perhaps advice, but are afraid of being pitied.

As they become more involved in the diagnostic and treatment regimens, they become more absorbed with their infertility. Their energy is sapped as they go from appointment to appointment and then try to find time to discuss the results and the implications with one another. Communication, sympathy, and understanding in the marriage become impaired. The strain on each partner's energy and self-esteem as well as on the marital system's energy reinforces the partners' isolation from one another and the world around them. Carol said, "I often felt I had to go somewhere and lick my wounds. I thought Bob was tired of hearing about everything, and my friends can only take so much, so I just tried to deal with a lot myself. I realized I was turning inward, but I didn't know what else to do."

Although others cannot feel the partners' stress or see the loss or the pain that contributes to their social isolation, they are real and overwhelming to both the partners and the couple system. These painful secrets further isolate the partners from one another and from friends and other supports.

Guilt

As they continue to struggle with their infertility problems, most partners also experience much guilt. They feel guilty because they cannot provide their partner with what he or she so desperately wants: the ability to fulfill the parental role. Perhaps they feel they have let down their parents or grandparents. As the role of parent appears dubious, they may feel guilty for being unable to carry out an important societal role that they see as a necessary aspect of contributing to their larger culture.

Some women feel guilt about previous sexual behavior. This is particularly true if the infertility problems seem related to scarring or obstructions from sexually transmitted diseases. Sadler and Syrop (1987) report that women with tubal disease feel guilty or punished by the infertility, whereas women experiencing endometriosis are more likely to feel helpless about their infertility.

Sometimes, difficulty conceiving or carrying a pregnancy can be related to damage from a previous abortion. Often the wife has tremendous difficulty discussing this guilt with her husband, or even admitting it, yet she suffers greatly. She feels she has been a bad person and has done some terrible things for which God is punishing her. Unfortunately, when struggling with the abortion issue, the wife's aloneness with this guilt further serves to isolate her with her pain.

If it is determined that one partner carries the impaired fertility, the other may feel resentment toward that partner, which may in turn create feelings of guilt. "I know it's not his fault; I mean, I know I shouldn't blame him," Carol cried during one session, "but sometimes I hate him for not being able to give me the child I want and then I feel so terribly guilty for hating him or for being angry." Sadler and Syrop (1987) report that in cases of male factor infertility, the wife often feels dissatisfied with sex and alternates between feelings of rage or protectiveness toward her husband. The fertile spouse attempts to rationalize a nonrational situation—to not feel the anger or resentment, which would be normal to feel. The ensuing guilt creates distance and isolation, further confounding the spouses' communication.

Depression and Grief

In the early stages of the couple's infertility experience there is no definitive explanation for their inability to conceive. As they look into an unknown future, they may feel loss similar to families experiencing the loss of a soldier missing in action (Sadler & Syrop, 1987). Such families do not have a clear explanation of what happened, do not know whether to give up hope, to have a funeral ritual, or to remain vigilant, but they know they feel a loss. There are no guarantees that they will obtain a definitive answer to resolve this loss, or find the reason—or the missing person—so they may remain in limbo for an indeterminate amount of time.

Ultimately the couple loses the fight; the spouses cannot function in denial or while feeling so angry or anxious. They begin to feel hopeless and depressed. The possibility of not achieving their role as biological parents begins to hit home. They feel hopeless regarding the viability of future treatments. They are tired and defeated and begin to lack the verve to continue fighting the uphill battle only to have their hopes dashed each month. They are losing energy for the issues and struggles of everyday life; they are losing their excitement for life and its meaning. "I don't feel excited by anything anymore," said Bob, who has always looked for the next challenge. "Nothing has meaning in my life. Maybe I need to do volunteer or charity work. Or maybe get involved in a church." He seemed puzzled about his lack of focus and meaning. Initially Bob attributed his malaise to a "mid-life crisis," but subsequently he realized it was related to not having the biological child about whom he'd always dreamed. "I feel I've lost my sense of purpose. I'm not sure what would bring meaning if I don't have a family," he explained during one session. "Life just seems so humdrum and sometimes bleak."

The depression isn't merely related to the loss of a biological child or the loss of the role of parent; it also encompasses the loss of the couple's dreams and fantasies of a child and family life. Often spouses have idealized the child and their family life. They fantasize a child more perfect than is realistically possible, family life that is beyond ordinary living (Sadler & Syrop, 1987). "Our childlessness creates a huge, gaping hole," Bob explained. Carol continued, "I can't imagine life without a child. I pictured us in the park. I pictured myself wheeling her in the stroller. I thought about those Christmas cards, you know, with the whole family pictured on the front? I just had so many plans." As already mentioned, the couple's loss experience is similar to a family dealing with chronic or terminal illness (McDaniel et al., 1992). So many plans are thwarted by the "illness," and a great despair is felt at the possibility of not being able to fulfill these plans.

Resolution

Healthy couples gradually move toward resolution. They learn how to cope: how to master, tolerate, or reduce the stress of the situation they feel exceeds their resources. They are gradually able to confront the situation and choose reality over denial (Callan & Hennessey, 1989). Ideally, the resolution will help them make peace with a specific choice about their family-building or guide them to choose child-free living. The turmoil they have been experiencing and the resulting threats to their relationship finally bring them face to face with one another to seek some type of truce in this overwhelming battle. However, resolution, particularly without psychotherapy, does not necessarily mean a couple "lives happily ever after." Some spouses divorce and eventually find other partners and have a family. Some spouses just move on, without making any definitive life plan or communicating about the trauma they experienced; they just continue to "exist," often remaining depressed, and plod through a life that holds little meaning. This is not a healthy resolution; it is merely a termination of treatment in an attempt to move on with life.

Until the partners have faced the loss of their dreams of being genetic parents or of nurturing a child, they cannot adequately resolve their infertility. They need to reevaluate their goals and their marriage. They need to again choose this partner over any other, even if it means not being able to become pregnant. Until they have accomplished this self-examination, they cannot complete the grief work that is mandatory for the resolution of infertility (Atwood & Dobkin, 1992; Sadler & Syrop, 1987). "I don't want to leave Bob, but I don't want to be childless, either," cried Carol during a particularly difficult session. "I just want us to make a decision. We need to talk about whether to try this last treatment or adopt. I don't want to keep ignoring this and leave it all just hanging unresolved."

Throughout a lifetime, many adults experience losses that precipitate depression, such as loss of status, self-esteem, health, confidence, fantasy fulfillment, and loss of someone of important symbolic value (Sadler & Syrop, 1987). Infertility involves all of these losses. However, as described above, the losses are invisible, and thus infertile couples are at risk for delayed or incomplete grief recovery.

In addition, the losses the infertile couple experience are not easily communicated The partners feel that their losses indicate a personal failure—that they are inadequate or defective or deviant. They do not want others to know these things for fear of being stigmatized. And because the loss is related to such a private part of their lives—their sexual functioning—they feel it is inappropriate to discuss their infertility issues with most friends and family members. Thus they may sacrifice these opportunities for support and become further isolated.

The monthly disappointments and feelings of loss are not acknowledged or validated by the larger society due to the secretiveness and invisible nature of the infertility losses. No one speaks of them or indicates a sensitivity to the devastation the couple experiences with the onset of each menstrual cycle. There are no socially acceptable avenues or rituals, such as a funeral service, to help them mourn. They are alone with their sorrow and pain. They suffer a special kind of grief that is unproclaimed and often misunderstood. Such unique aspects of the infertility experiences make it difficult for these couples to resolve their grief.

Problems with the Sexual Relationship

Infertility is often the first crisis the couple encounters. It tests the partners' ability to communicate and threatens their sexuality. As McDaniel and colleagues (1992) state, "Diagnosis and treatment of infertility result in a major invasion of privacy in the most intimate area of a couple's relationship, their sex life." Since it is not merely a physical condition, but an emotional and social one as well, it requires a great commitment of resources by the couple.

Other than the loss of control and monthly sense of failure, a partner may exhibit somatic reactions, such as headaches and stomach or intestinal problems, which can reinforce sexual insecurities and doubts (McDaniel et al., 1992). When infertility is attributed to male factor difficulties, men become impotent in about 80 percent of the cases (Sadler & Syrop, 1987). Bob talked about his feelings of not being sexually adequate and his fears of not being sexually attractive to Carol or other women. Because their infertility problems were attributed to male factor problems, he felt his body was out of control and he began to question his sexual potency. "I feel so inadequate. I just don't feel virile or powerful these days and I can't imagine that Carol sees me that way either. I'm sure that accounts for the lack of interest in our lovemaking." Women with ovulatory dysfunction experience poor body image and therefore a sense of decreased sexual desirability. Understandably, they also report poor self-esteem and feelings of inadequacy (Sadler & Syrop, 1987).

Sexual intercourse can become aversive when it is "on demand" in order to accommodate the fertile part of the cycle. Intercourse may be uncomfortable because of the side effects of hormone injections or physical reactions to medication. The couple's sexual functions are particularly sensitive to the stressors of the infertility. In their research, Berg and Wilson (1991) found that the longer the couple had been in treatment, the lower their levels of sexual satisfaction. However, their research also indicated that most indices of sexual functioning, such as levels of desire, frequency, or erectile and ejaculatory difficulties, did not vary through the years of treatment. Other research has reported that, as a response to the stress of treatment and decreased levels of satisfaction, one or both partners may engage in affairs, sexually seductive behaviors, or other ways of sexually acting out (Butler & Koraleski, 1990; Callan & Hennessey, 1989).

Long-Term Effects

Unfortunately, the feelings experienced during the course of the diagnostic tests and medical treatments do not simply disappear when the couple achieves pregnancy or some other type of resolution. The effects of the infertility diagnosis and treatments over a protracted time period produce negative psychological consequences. In their research with infertile couples extending over a three-year period, Berg and Wilson (1991) found that during the first year of infertility treatment couples perceived their marital adjustment and sexual relationship as adequate, but that the acute stress of beginning treatments had started to affect each individual's psychological functioning. During the second year of treatment, psychological functioning was still within normal limits. The most dramatic difficulties occurred during the third year of treatment. Couples reported increased psychological strain, depression, marital strain, and, often, increases in hostility, anxiety, and obsessive-compulsive behaviors. As with any crisis, the functional impairments were of lasting duration. The negative feelings about one's body image, the emotional scars of the monthly cycle of loss, or the anxiety of living childless did not quickly dissipate, regardless of the type of resolution the couple reached.

The medical diagnosis of infertility manifests no outward physical symptoms or blemishes, yet the partners are impaired and feel defective. Since an individual's identity is shaped around his or her sense of body image, physical well-being, and intactness (Sadler &

Syrop, 1987), these individuals have negative feelings about their bodies and perceive their bodies as having betrayed them. Women are particularly susceptible to feelings of negative self-image since our society places a premium on the perfect body, beautiful hair, and youthful vibrancy (Butler & Koraleski, 1990). The additional burden, of course, is the societal pressure to become a mother through pregnancy and childbirth. Faced with an inability or difficulty in carrying out this injunction, women may turn their negative feelings inward and exhibit self-hatred. This may manifest through overeating or poor grooming. These feelings of negativity or failure may be further exacerbated by feelings of lack of control, exhibited through obsessive behaviors or anorexic or bulimic behaviors. Through such behaviors she hopes to gain some control, but the behavior verifies the lack of regard for her body.

When an individual is in crisis, he or she experiences difficulties in cognitive functioning such as the inability to focus, disorganization, a decrease of thought processes, and fatigue. Couples experiencing infertility describe a sense of unfairness, unfulfillment, and disappointment (Valentine, 1986). Efforts to control, such as developing obsessions, may serve as coping mechanisms, but are not successful mechanisms in terms of the marital relationship. In fact, these behaviors put more strain on the marriage, and cause an isolated couple to become more emotionally fragile (Valentine, 1986). The intensity and lasting duration of the infertility experience create chronic stress for the couple. As discussed previously, infertility affects not only each individual, but the marital system and sexual relationship as well (Berg & Wilson, 1991). And because the crisis of infertility is pervasive and so extensive, the partners experience reverberations throughout their lives. There may be frequent painful reminders, even when they believe their infertility has been resolved. They may be especially aware during holiday or birthday times, when they have no child to share the experience with. Or they may feel especially empty at the death of a close family member, as they see their family dwindling with no new members to carry on. Or they may have an especially anxious pregnancy and respond in overprotective ways toward the child they do ultimately conceive. Adoptive couples may grieve the pregnancy they didn't experience as well as the continued loss of their biological heritage. "We are so glad that we were able to finally move on and adopt. We are crazy about our little guy. But you know there are still difficult times," explained Bob, when he and Carol came for a follow-up session. "I was actually surprised," continued Carol. "I thought we had done such a good job of resolving our infertility, and I thought adopting Michael would be the final stage of moving on. But then my cousin got pregnant on her third in vitro attempt. It has been so hard. I am happy for her because I know what she's been through, and yet I'm sad and jealous because she gets to experience all the pregnancy stuff."

Emotional Healing

Couples find a number of ways to adapt to the crisis of infertility. Some manage a controlled reaction in order to gradually expose themselves to the reality. Some rage explosively. Some spouses may actively express anger with each other, their doctors, or fate. Some couples alternate between these reactions (Callan & Hennessey, 1989).

Spouses may seek psychotherapy at any of several junctures:

- They begin to realize the extent of their pain and how it has interrupted their life plan and their relationship.
- They begin to recognize that the infertility has taken over their lives, their communication, and their marriage.
- They begin to comprehend the extent to which their intense focus has isolated them from family, social activities, and even each other.
- They see that it is a problem that will not go away.
- They begin to experience reminders or they overreact to a friend's comment, a pregnancy, baby shower, or even a wedding.
- They are aware of encountering something larger, more consuming, and more encompassing than any other obstacle they have probably experienced.

When a couple initially enters therapy, the partners are confused and overwhelmed. They are feeling powerful emotions and may even be experiencing intense emotional ups and downs. Therefore, during the initial stage of therapy, the therapist reminds them that many of their feelings are typical of individuals in crisis. The emphasis needs to be on education. The therapist must teach them about the medical process, the drug side effects, and the prolonged psychological stress they will experience. This way, the partners can begin to piece together a context—a picture of the mountain they are about to attempt to climb.

During the second phase of psychotherapy, the therapist will help the partners focus on issues surrounding their social functioning. They must make many decisions regarding how long to continue treatment, whom to tell, and how much to tell. Should they tell their families why they are participating less in family functions? Why they opted to vacation during Christmas rather than attend the traditional family celebration? Their decisions about how long to continue treatment and what and when to explain to family or office coworkers have consequences for career and other life goals.

As the medical treatments continue and become more involved, the couple reaches more difficult decision points. The complex technology and the emphasis on decision-making around issues of medical and moral questions specific to infertility further complicate this emotionally laden crisis. So in the third phase of psychotherapy the couple is forced to struggle with the degree of effectiveness of the various assisted reproductive technologies, such as in vitro fertilization (IVF) or gamete intra-fallopian transfer (GIFT). In addition, the couple may have to struggle with religious sanctions against these procedures or their own moral codes that challenge questions about life and its origins.

The Initial Stage of Psychotherapy

In the initial stage of therapy, the therapist must immediately begin to normalize the couple's experiences. The spouses need reassurance that infertility is a medical and physical problem that greatly affects psychological functioning—it is not a flaw in their character or a psychologically generated problem. In many cases, the couple has not been educated about the side effects of the infertility drugs. Often physicians are so familiar with the medications they prescribe that they minimally, if at all, address the psychological or emotional impact of the treatments, or sometimes they believe such information does not belong in the medical office. The therapist should educate the couple if appropriate and, above all, validate that the couple is indeed reacting to powerful drugs that have various side effects. The interaction of synthetic or natural hormones with an intense emotional issue will generate powerful reactions; moodiness or emotional outbursts are common. When spouses become educated regarding the enormous extent of the drugs' effects and understand how normal the intensity of their emotions really is, the cycles—and their lives—become more manageable.

At this point, the therapist can review or teach crisis intervention strategies in order to help the couple cope with the intense reactions to the acute strain of infertility. These reactions can manifest in psychological and sexual symptoms (Berg & Wilson, 1991). Reactions that become chronic will require more intensive intervention; at this initial stage, however, crisis intervention stategies are quite useful since many of the couple's behavioral reactions are similar to those experienced by people in crisis. Valentine (1986) defines a crisis as a period of disorganization followed by an intense preoccupation with a specific event. Valentine also reports that 10 of the 14 couples she interviewed described their experience as an obsession with infertility—that is, a preoccupation with the situation.

Helping couples cope means helping them accept and redefine their situation. A way for the therapist to do this would be to suggest support or RESOLVE groups. Knowing that others have similar problems helps the couple feel less weird and isolated. Through talking with others in support groups or RESOLVE groups, the partners begin to perceive their feelings as normal. If they can positively compare their situation to others', even if only to say they have at least found a cause for their infertility, they can improve their coping abilities (Callan & Hennessey, 1989). This was true for Bob and Carol. As they struggled in one therapy session to make sense of the exhausting diagnostic tests, Carol said, "I'm so glad you told us to go to that support group. It really helped to hear others say exactly what *I* was feeling. I didn't feel so weird. And I'm so glad we're almost at the end of these tests. One woman in the group said things got easier once they knew what their problem was and how to fix it. Our medical team already has some ideas about what our problems might be. So I'm feeling more hopeful now."

The therapist should also help the couple devise other coping strategies; Callan and Hennessey (1989) have noted that the more strategies partners have, the more protected they seem to be from the effects of psychological stress. The partners need help learning to have fun again, encouragement to develop various interests and distractions, and suggestions for planning activities as well as social occasions.

The therapist will also help the partners construct a new world view (Atwood & Dobkin, 1992), one that is more congruent with their infertility experiences. They must be pushed to challenge their present thinking by asking new questions, thus opening new doors. They must search for meaning from their negative experience. They need to create a psychological transition, since the infertility "constitutes a deconstruction of the anticipatory role of biological parent and the construction of a new identity consonant with the infertility information, which for many is psychologically the most difficult and stressful undertaking of the grieving process" (Atwood & Dobkin, 1992, p. 393). Specific questions can help the couple search for meaning:

- If they look at their relationship prior to the infertility crisis, what do they see? Who were they, as indiviuals and as a couple?
- If they examine their coping patterns prior to their infertility crisis, can they find coping mechanisms and old strengths that may serve well today?
- If they want to enjoy life more, and one another, what do they need to do differently?
- If their discussions were not so burdened with infertility-related issues, what else would they want to talk about?
- What hobbies/interests have they always wanted to pursue, individually or together, that would be challenging as well fulfilling? What do they need to do in order to accomplish them?

They need to allow compassion and forgiveness for oneself as well as the partner. They need to discuss ways to take a more active role in their life decisions and to let go of their anger about their lack of control. These questions and discussions can help the partners reframe the crisis and the all-encompassing nature of the infertility experience. It is important that they believe they are doing all they can throughout the process.

In the following dialogue, Bob and Carol express their struggle as they attempt to make the psychological transition.

Carol: So one day I just decided I was tired of feeling sad, tired of feeling like everyone else was dictating what I needed to do. I remembered that I always used to be the one in charge, and that I still am that person in my office. I just need to become that person again at home and in the doctor's office. It was helpful to think about all the questions you posed last session.

Therapist: I'm glad you found it useful to look at who you were before all of the infertility trauma and to look at what you were doing and what you found rewarding in your life prior to this crisis. Which questions from last session did you find particularly helpful for you, Carol?

Carol: Well, when you asked about my life goals and how having a child fit into those, I remembered that in fact I did have other life goals, I always have. I became so consumed by this baby-making stuff that I practically forgot that other things have meaning in my life too. I was thinking how much I like to travel. I reminded Bob that we've put so much of our life on hold—we even stopped planning trips. I'd like to travel again. I also thought about taking those flute lessons I've always had my heart set on. All those questions you asked gave me pause and pushed me to finally look at myself and my direction in a new way.

Bob: When I saw Carol examining all of this, I thought, hey, I'm okay too. She's right, we've let so much go in our lives. We stopped hoping and reaching out for adventure and new challenges. That's just not me, but I want it to be me again. And I want it to be us. There was a way in which we used to push each other; if she would dare, I would do it, and vice versa. I want that back again!

As the infertility treatments continue over time, couples' coping mechanisms become strained. The crisis intervention techniques discussed above are no longer adequate to bring relief. Chronic strain reactions require different types of psychological intervention (Berg & Wilson, 1991). The infertility experience may also open other unresolved conflicts for the individuals or the couple system, and may even create other psychological symptoms, such as agoraphobia or other anxiety reactions, eating disorders, or depression, so that more intensive intervention is required.

The Second Stage of Psychotherapy

In the second stage of psychotherapy, the therapist must first assess whether a more serious psychological disorder, such as a panic or eating disorder, has developed as a result of the infertility crisis. Such a disorder must be dealt with specifically, in an intense and direct manner, prior to a more complete focus on the infertility issues per se. Such dysfunction hinders individual functioning, decision-making, and even one's physical and psychological health. Therefore, the resolution of any such disorder is the first and immediate focal point of therapy.

In the second stage of psychotherapy, the therapist should also continue to

- encourage the partners to express and acknowledge their anger, disappointment, and any other intense emotions they have been experiencing, and
- validate these feelings, thus normalizing the experience and helping the couple feel more in control.

During this stage, the therapist will also assist the partners in separating their sexuality, self-image, and self-esteem from the childbearing issue (Sadler & Syrop, 1987). There may have been shifts in the power structure or decision-making processes between them as they struggled with their infertility. These dynamics should be reassessed to determine whether they are currently healthy and adaptive for the couple.

The marital system often needs rebalancing in order to ensure that the infertility is defined as a *couple's* issue. This involves reexamining the marital boundaries since they may have become too centered around a desired child. Here are some questions the therapist should consider:

- Has the infertility and the childless state become the "identified patients," the focal point of all the couple's problems and troubles?
- Have the partners become triangulated around the anticipated child, thus losing the connection with one another?
- Have the partners isolated from their extended family and friends?

The partners need to understand that their marital system is stressed and needs attention. As a way of recovering from the infertility crisis, they must reconnect with their supports and decrease their level of secrecy and isolation. Callan and Hennessey (1989) have found evidence of a connection between social support from friends and family and better recovery from stressful life events. Such reconnection involves conscious decisions about the extent of involvement with extended family—whom to tell and how much to tell—and how to establish new boundaries. To this end, the therapist will aid the partners in deciding what to share with others and how to handle specific situations with family, friends, and coworkers. This includes identifying those who may offer comfort, those who could help them further clarify their feelings or goals, and those who may positively challenge them in order to help them work through decisions (Williams, Bischoff, & Ludes, 1992).

Once these decisions have been made, the partners may want to instruct these significant people in their lives regarding how to interact more sensitively with them. The therapist may guide them through role play in order to practice communication skills. Acting out various situations or discussions with family or friends will help the couple become more confident with the actual behaviors.

The process outlined above will help the partners strengthen their marital system and define themselves in ways they probably never had prior to this crisis. It will also push them to be more aware of their goals, their adaptation to one another, and how they function in crisis. The therapy continues with a reassessment of the couple's system dynamics, a reframing of the infertility experience as a developmental crisis. As Bob and Carol explained, they needed to stop defining themselves as infertile people.

Bob: Because I thought of myself as infertile, I labeled myself defective. I forgot I was a very good hospital administrator, a good athlete, and [he laughs] even a good husband. I forgot I had all these other parts to me.

Therapist: You need to frequently recollect all of these other very functional parts of yourself, Bob, because you need to keep track of the context of your whole self, your whole life, not just this narrow window you two have looked through lately. I think you started to see your life in black and white instead of color. You and Carol also became two people walking along parallel paths instead of a team working through an isolated crisis together. You have encountered a developmental hurdle. Don't get confused and think you have become weird or defective.

Carol: You know, you're right. That's exactly what happened. We both thought we were weird and so we hid, we got so isolated, probably to hide from ourselves as well as each other. Because I was disappointed in our lives, at least our nonparenting lives, I generalized that to being disappointed in Bob too. I forgot that we are both such vibrant people. We became 1-D instead of 3-D [she laughs].

Therapist: It's so good that you both can see how you inadvertently strayed down this path—and how you can return to where you were before. More importantly, you are beginning to see that you two have not changed, but rather the circumstances of your life transported you to a place you didn't understand and had no way to interpret, so you assumed it meant you were inadequate to conquer it or to move beyond it. Now you are beginning to build on your assets and create a perspective in order to make some sense of this crisis.

The emphasis in this second stage of therapy is on assessing and revitalizing the marital relationship, since in the earlier infertility experience the partners focused on the crisis, their loss, and the negative aspects of their lives. In the third stage of therapy they will need to renew their strength and vitality individually and as a couple in order to make difficult decisions about their continued treatment.

The Third Stage of Psychotherapy

During the final stage of therapy, the therapist will continue to help the spouses explore tools that will help them move past this crisis. Discussions will focus on their roles, communication patterns, and life goals, as well as their desires for a child and for parenting, which may be different for each partner. Although this may seem overwhelming to the couple, when divided into smaller manageable steps, the process becomes useful and often healing.

Assisting the partners in developing a plan and setting goals is also important, because it helps them once again feel some sense of control over their lives. To escape feeling "betrayed by their bodies, victimized by their treatments, and totally at the mercy of their doctors and fate" (Butler & Koraleski, 1990), they need to determine where they can relinquish control and in what areas they can exert control while accepting the limits they have regarding control over their physiology. Their medical treatment goals should be established within the context of these physiological limits. By examining the control they can have over other life options and goals, they can then begin making specific plans to accomplish some of these other life goals. These goals may be career-related, such as pursuing further education or a more challenging job, or related to the couple's lifestyle, such as buying a new home, a vacation home, or planning a second honeymoon or other exciting travel. Their planning should be focused on finding ways to make their lives meaningful and productive again.

There are several tools the therapist can use to aid the discussions around this goal-setting.

1. Help the partners create a decision balance sheet where they identify their feelings and the pros and cons of the goals they are exploring.
2. Guided imagery exercises can help the spouses clarify their

desires. Have them imagine their career, vacations, leisure time, and other lifestyle considerations, both with and without a child.

3. Suggest that each partner keep a journal that allows for the free flow of expression, feelings, and processing of the therapy; such a journal can help each individual clarify his or her thinking.

4. As in the first stage of therapy, encourage the partners to talk with other couples who are going through the infertility experience, who can help them see that many of their reactions are common, and from whom they may learn of alternate avenues for the pursuit of parenting. Attending RESOLVE meetings, particularly the support group meetings, can be a good source for meeting others struggling with these same issues. The RESOLVE meeting context also allows the partners to feel they are helping others deal with their infertility, which raises their self-esteem and increases their coping abilities (Callan & Henessey, 1989).

5. Teach techniques for stress management and conflict resolution. If the partners can reduce their stress and anxiety, they will be better able to handle the continued medical procedures and the ups and downs of the monthly cycle, and to think more clearly and work through the issues. Relaxation and assertiveness communication skills are particularly useful. Conflict resolution techniques will ease the partners' struggle to heal relationships with their families and larger social networks. Such techniques further help them heal their own relationship as they sort through their differences and examine what might be more realistic to expect from one another. Learning to listen, paraphrase, and then respond without defensiveness enable the partners to realize they can confront and resolve differences.

6. If appropriate, urge the partners to set limits around the amount of time each day they can discuss their infertility. Partners frequently have different needs regarding the discussion of their infertility and the options. Making a pact to limit their discussions to 20 or 30 minutes a day, for example, during which each would tell their concerns,

questions, and feelings, allows them to explore other facets of their relationship at other times. This technique pushes them to relate as a couple, not just an infertile couple.

7. Recommend a more extensive time-out if necessary—a "vacation" from treatments. The couple may need the psychological and physical space from the monthly grind in order to gain some perspective. This break can help the partners see how large the infertility looms in their lives, and thus its impact on their communication, their sexual interaction, their careers and their lives.

8. As the spouses get back in touch with one another, encourage a return to play and romance. After focusing so long on "baby-making," they now need permission to return to love-making. Creating romantic interludes could be a good beginning for them to become reinvolved in more recreational, fun, and passionate sexual interactions.

Bob and Carol talked about how some of these tools improved their communication with each other and changed their views of the future.

Bob: Your idea to take this month off turned out to be a good thing. Carol's body needed a rest, but so did we! I realized that even when we weren't talking about our infertility she was up in the bedroom reading about it. If I said something, she'd just say, "What do you care? I'm not bothering you with all this." So I was relieved when we had the forced break because we learned to do other things and talk about other things—even fun things like where to take vacation!

Therapist: It's good you realized how easy it was to become consumed by your discussions around the infertility. You have been working harder, Bob, to really listen and not jump in and try to fix it or to get impatient with Carol.

Carol: Yes, the paraphrasing you taught us has helped a lot. But I've also been trying to really focus my complaining or my anger into those 20 minutes. And at other times I've really worked to think about just how much further I want to go with all this.

Therapist: That is certainly important for you to begin thinking about Carol, but you *both* need to begin talking about that too. Bob has been expressing his thoughts about stopping mostly because he worries about what you're going through. You may not be as ready to stop, but you do need to let him know where you stand. And both of you need to remember to use those communication skills we've been practicing here.

Elected vacations from treatment or enforced rests often evolve into a decision to cease treatments. What makes it difficult for many couples to decisively end treatment is the lack of a distinct medical ending point as well as their own ambivalence. "I don't know how much longer I can go through all of this," Carol cried during one of the following sessions, "and I know it's so hard on Bob, but there seems to always be one more procedure, one more hope. It makes it so difficult to just give up on my hope for a biological child and my hope to be pregnant." Often there is no clear point where couples believe they have exhausted all their options. Most couples have indicated they would rather be told conclusively that there is no chance of pregnancy than hold onto hope when there is a poor prognosis (Berg & Wilson, 1991).

The therapist can help the partners decide when to end treatment by discussing a time frame and some limits for medical treatment. They need to sense that treatment does not have to go on forever and be able to make informed decisions. Directing them to places they can obtain information about up-to-date medical interventions and options, as well as other alternatives, can be quite useful at this point.

In order to work from an informed stance, they need to understand the facts of their situation, how optimistic or hopeless it really is. They need to challenge their medical team with the information they are learning. It is useful to rehearse ways of working with their medical providers through discussion and role play in order to encourage a free flow of information (McDaniel et al., 1992).

A large part of the problem for couples is that assisted reproductive technologies continue to advance in sophistication and specialty, which makes it harder to let go. However, the procedures are more complex and demanding and require "substantial increments in time, expense, physical involvement, and emotional stress, coupled with very low success rates and potential moral dilemmas involving the technology" (Berg & Wilson, 1991, p. 23). The process of exploring and discussing the various options is exhausting. The partners see the decision-making process as crucial and as serious as a life-death decision. Because their parenthood is threatened, their marriage itself is threatened, which exerts further pressure.

At some point the partners must face the necessity of moving on with their lives. Often, the trigger for stopping treatment is not sensational, but nonetheless provokes the turning point. It may be a comment from a friend, too much frustration with the conflicts over treatment and career schedules, or even the realization that they just don't have the energy for yet another cycle of human menopausal gonadotropins (e.g., Fertinex) or IVF or temperature-taking.

Eventually, and often with the assistance of psychotherapy, they are able to accept their infertility and move on with life. However, as Diane Cole (1988) poignantly explains, accepting one's infertility "entails first a surrendering of possibility, the tossing off of a dream that one has dreamed for many years. And the death of that dream means finding a way to define oneself anew, to peer into the future and imagine a different self, a different life, a different family, a family of two, and maybe someday one" (page 65). The partners need to examine the consequences of their intense focus on pregnancy and reexamine their decisions and priorities. They must rework their dream and find meaning in other aspects of their lives. They must discover their own resolution and begin to move toward those goals.

During the final stage of therapy, the therapist helps the couple construct a resolution (Atwood & Dobkin, 1992). How important is parenting at this time? What are the couple's options for parenting? Although the partners need not let go of the idea of parenting, they do need to let go of their dream of a biological child. They need to acknowledge their fantasies and then begin the grieving process for this child. This may involve ceremonies, rituals, or just discussing these fantasies with one another. They may want to write a letter to this imagined child, telling her of all the special activities they had planned. They may want to designate a particular place at or near their home where this child would "reside." The couple may want to tell one another or other family members their sadness about this fantasized child's special eyes, just like Dad's, or special musical talent, just like Mom's.

The couple may also grieve the actual pregnancy experience, of feeling the baby kick, having others ask about the pregnancy, or seeing the baby on the ultrasound. The partners need to begin to explore the concept of parenthood in an entirely new context.

The couple now needs to look to the future. How do the partners envision this future? Is a child involved? Is parenthood still a goal? What do their values and religious and ethical views tell them about their future course? What about their career goals? How do these fit into the larger picture of life goals? And how do all of these issues impact the decision around a child and raising that child?

When the partners can separate the concept of pregnancy from their ultimate goal of parenting, they can then more easily grieve the pregnancy and a biological child. Then they can more readily project into their future. As the therapist reviews each partner's needs and values, they can begin to communicate the issues they dared not think about or discuss while undergoing the medical interventions. As they have been told in other stages of their infertility, they may not be in the same place at the same time; they may not be ready for a certain option together. However, communication about their process is important to work their way out of the crises of infertility. This is a step-by-step process, often painful, but necessary in order to resolve their infertility. When working through such pain and sorrow, the process of resolution will bring them closer to one another and to their ultimate goal, whether that be parenting or child-free living.

4

THE IMPACT OF GENDER
IN DEALING WITH
INFERTILITY ISSUES

THE CHALLENGES AND DISAPPOINTMENTS of infertility are experienced, interpreted, and managed differently by each individual in the couple relationship. Although some of the variability can be attributed to differences in personality, life experiences, or even one's role and experience in the family of origin, a major factor accounting for unique reactions to the infertility experience is gender. Unfortunately, gender often serves to magnify the pain and confusion experienced by both partners.

"Jason doesn't understand me," Lisa complained during one therapy session. "He never did and now it seems worse with all of these infertility issues. We just seem to speak a different language or something. Sometimes I wonder if we've been in the same room with the same doctors." Lisa's frustration about their different perceptions reflects an age-old dilemma written and spoken about by both men and women. References to infertility and men and women's distinct reactions to the experience date as far back as the biblical story of Hannah. Hannah's husband, Elkanah, "feeling helpless and desperate to make her happier, attempts to use logic to help her feel better. Like many of today's husbands, he cannot understand why his love of her, and the special attention he gives her, is not enough to make her happy" (Cooper & Glazer, 1994, p. 4).

The complexity of the infertility experience is magnified by the inherent complexity of gender differences. Because husbands and wives experience infertility differently, they are puzzled as to how to help and support one another. Even if spouses are able to comfort each other during the difficult circumstances of an illness, "infertility cannot be treated like other illnesses because it deals with the essence of maleness and femaleness" (Sadler & Syrop, 1987, p. 8).

The Influence of Gender on Viewing Infertility

The Commonalities of Men's and Women's Views on Infertility

Typically, more attention has been given to gender differences than to similarities, although the empirical findings are mixed regarding the existence of gender differences in psychological functioning (Berg, Wilson, & Weingartner, 1991). Men and women often struggle—and fight—about what they perceive to be differences in reactions. "When we realized we might be infertile, I cried and cried," Lisa explained during one particularly emotional session. "Jason just stood there and said we should consider other options. He was so unemotional." Jason quickly defended himself, "I just didn't know what to do. Good old competent Lisa was falling apart before my eyes. I just felt I had to find an answer, some hope. I was scared and disappointed too."

For different reasons, the diagnostic process is just as problematic for men as it is for women. For both, the importance of having a child increases after the infertility diagnosis (Berg et al., 1991). It would seem that as the couple faces the prospect of childlessness, both partners confront the reality of an emotional void in their lives. All of their fears and questions may not seem real until they actually hear the diagnosis from their doctors. Both partners experience a sinking feeling as they face the disappointment, the loss of their fantasies, and the prospect of childlessness. Both partners experience pain. Since this pain involves a major life issue, it transcends their present experience; it is probably the first time they have faced a threat to their adequacy and self-esteem.

An important aspect of their distress is its context, which usually involves their life pursuits or goals. Stanton, Tennen, Affleck, and Mendola (1991) report that 61 percent of the women in their study and 49 percent of the men reported feeling that infertility threatened important life goals. Gretchen, a 35-year-old school principal, explained, "I am so angry. I am used to doing whatever I please and having my life the way I want it. Now I'm at the mercy of the medical team; they tell me I can't even exercise during these treatments. Despite all of these treatments, I don't even have the family I want. I don't see an end to this. I don't know how we will achieve our dream."

Her husband, Steven, added, "I thought I would get my dental practice started, start having our kids, and then kind of take it easy. I had dreams about using those school vacations that Gretchen and the kids would have to go skiing, to Disney World, or to our summer home. I'm at a loss now. My practice is doing well, but I don't know what else to do with my life."

Female Reactions to Infertility

RESPONSE TO MEDICAL TREATMENT

Historically, infertility has been viewed as a female problem, both in the physical and psychological domains. Individuals tend to accept that much of their distress is due to gender differences. However, a major cause of these different reactions between the male and female might well be the different degree of treatment-related stress that each suffers. Generally, the medical process is far more invasive and stressful for the woman. Often, it is the way in which women are treated during this process, rather than the occurrence of infertility itself, that leads to the disparity of reactions between a man and a woman. It should be kept in mind, therefore, that some of what may be interpreted as gender differences may in fact be explained as women's reactions to the extensive medical interventions. Women's experience as the focus of treatment sets up dynamics that label them as patients. Thus, issues around self-concept and self-deprecation often arise as a result of an infertility work-up.

Women are more accustomed to seeking routine reproductive health care and are therefore the most likely to initially suspect infertility and arrange the first medical contact (Berg et al., 1991; Newton & Houle, 1993; Sadler & Syrop, 1987). Women are also more likely to engage in infertility-related activities, such as reading about it or talking to professionals or to other couples. Additionally, because of their greater likelihood of involvement in medical systems, women have had a greater number of medical procedures available to them and thus have been more involved in the medical procedures (Stanton, Tennen, Affleck, & Mendola, 1991).

Since women visit medical offices more frequently than men, they are more available for research, so that more is known and reported about women's reactions and experience. According to Burns (1993), anxiety and major depressive episodes are the most commonly diagnosed psychiatric problems among those experiencing infertility, especially women. However, if women are more usually the focus of research, do such results really indicate that women suffer these psychiatric difficulties to a greater degree than men? Other research indicates that although women show greater variability in emotional responses (Newton & Houle, 1993), significant emotional maladjustment is no more prevalent in women coping with infertility than for the general population of women (Paulson, Haarmann, Salerno, & Asmar, 1988). Whether men and women suffer in a like manner and whether men and women who experience infertility suffer more or differently than the general population are areas that need further research. However, the research also needs to neutralize gender bias by targeting both men's and women's issues more equitably and to explain differences in reactions within the context of differences in how the genders respond, rather than attributing reactions necessarily to differences in feelings.

Even if some of the gender differences reported are related to investigative methods, research indicates that women are initially more affected than men when the inability to conceive is first noted (Newton & Houle, 1993). Because the infertility experience rocks the central core of a woman, she is more likely to openly discuss her distress and to look for support and solutions such as medical treatment or counseling. If children are more important to the wife, Abbey, Andrews, and Halman (1991) report that she feels more disruption and stress in the couple's personal, social, and sex lives. The disruption and disappointment cause women to experience depressive symptoms, even in the early stages of medical treatment. As women continue through treatments, the depression increases with a concomitant decrease in self-esteem (Newton & Houle, 1993).

RESPONSE TO PROGNOSIS

The inherent uncertainty about the causes, treatments, and prognosis also contributes to a sense of ambiguity in the lives of infertile women; women experience uncertainty about their identity and their life pursuits (Sandelowski, 1987, p. 70). This situation forces women to continually construct and reconstruct their reality and their identities. "Women's efforts to reduce ambiguity also [lead] them to search for ultimate causes by juxtaposing science with religion, the rational with the irrational, and the temporal with the spiritual" (Sandelowski, 1987, p. 72). As Gretchen summarized, "I keep telling myself I have so much else in my life. I am respected and liked. I have a good career path, perhaps even becoming the superintendent. But I wonder, if I weren't so successful—and so stressed—would I be more likely to become pregnant? If I weren't so lucky to be working around kids all the time, would I be rewarded by having my own child because I wouldn't have kids in my life? I know it's stupid, but I can't help sometimes thinking that way."

Infertility treatments require women to intently observe and document their bodies, often on a daily basis. This heightens the degree of involvement by a woman in the diagnostic process and increases her feelings of responsibility. As she becomes sensitive to the nuances of her body, she spends much time and energy monitoring her body, particularly for signs of pregnancy. Such close scrutiny contributes to a sense of loss of control. Ironically, however, the more helpless she feels, the more responsibility she assumes for her and her husband's failed attempts.

Women seem to blame themselves no matter what the cause of the infertility (Berg et al., 1991; McEwan et al., 1987; Newton & Houle, 1993). They are more likely to assume personal responsibility even after a male factor diagnosis has been made. Interestingly, the women indicated feeling punished regardless of whose factor created the infertility. Sometimes wives even reported claiming the infertility problem when it was clearly related to the husband's factors.

Infertility prompts women to reexamine their lifestyles, careers, and major life goals. Sometimes they attempt lifestyle changes, such as an increase or decrease in physical activity, or they may leave a challenging job, thinking that will allow for developing other interests or perhaps reduce stess enough to more easily become pregnant. The net result is merely further reduction in their quality of life. Younger women experience more distress with their infertility and restricted life options, possibly because women who waited longer were more involved in other areas of their lives and therefore do not have so much invested in one arena of their functioning.

EFFECT ON CAREER
The infertility crisis affects careers in different ways. Many women hold onto a job while waiting to get pregnant, intending to leave or work part-time in order to provide childcare. Sometimes a woman holds onto a job or career for fear of making a change to a new employer who won't understand the crisis she is going through, or because she needs that medical insurance. Or she may hold on because it is a source of self-esteem or even diversion from the pain of the infertility. "Yet even women who have been highly successful in their careers . . . feel a tremendous gap in their lives when they . . . discover they are infertile" (Cooper & Glazer, 1994, p. 11). In fact, it may be somewhat misleading for women who desire children to assume they can find adequate compensations for childlessness. Certainly their careers or changes in their careers may not be sufficient to absorb the disappointment.

Male Reactions to Infertility

The way infertility affects men may be more subtle and therefore not as easily measured with our current research methods or not as readily labeled within our cultural contexts. Additionally, "because society does not support men expressing their emotions or claiming ownership of their role in reproduction, some men may be out of touch or secretive about infertility and their distress may be missed" (McDaniel et al., 1992). Although most men seem to react with less emotional distress than women, it may be that their distress is more covert. Perhaps their perceived differences are related to the fact that men have different coping mechanisms and are better at compartmentalizing their feelings or are more likely to engage in strategies of distancing or self-control (Newton & Houle, 1993). Husbands report that they have the most difficulty dealing with their wife's pain; although they may appear to be larely unaffected by the crisis, they may be utilizing strategies of self-control or distancing in order to be strong for their wives (Berg et al., 1991; McDaniel et al., 1992; Newton & Houle, 1993). Men may withdraw emotionally because they are helpless to fix the pain; their lack of communication about the issues may be an attempt to protect their partner from the pain. In the research conducted by Valentine (1986), men reported wanting to be more supportive through discussing the infertility but indicated this increased their stress.

While men and women experience similar feelings of worry, tension, irritation, and sadness, Berg and Wilson (1990) report that men experience these feelings less frequently. Men may also be more likely to label their feelings as frustration and anger (Sadler & Syrop, 1987) when in fact they may be feelings of loss they are experiencing. The primary concerns for a man are the loss of his mate and the fear she'll never return to her previous self.

Jeremy, a successful college professor, was able to articulate his pain regarding this loss: "I am so useless with Emily's pain. We go to a store, a restaurant—I never know where it will happen—and she sees a baby or child and starts to cry. I just don't know when it will happen or what to do to comfort her. I get so I hate to go out with her because I just don't know what to do. She's just not the same person. I don't know how to talk to her or how to comfort her. She told me I used to be her best friend and now I don't feel like any kind of friend."

Lisa's husband, Jason, explained his frustration and helplessness as he watched Lisa struggle with her lack of control over their fertility. "Lisa seems unfocused and so dejected much of the time," Jason complained during one therapy session. "She puts herself down a lot and she's so wrapped up with what's going on with her body. I hate losing her this way."

"Men, who are used to being in control and being able to use logic and reasoning to solve problems, may feel useless" (Cooper & Glazer, 1994). Like Jeremy, they may feel helpless. The helplessness is so intolerable that they may withdraw emotionally, leaving their wives feeling abandoned and alone in their crisis. In therapy, Emily revealed that she was certain Jeremy didn't understand her; she even questioned whether he really desired a child. Because he was more apt to use logic and try to fix the situation, Jeremy was more focused on a solution, such as an end to the treatment. This further fueled Emily's fears that he didn't desire a child or at least didn't desire one to the same degree. She wondered if they were still in agreement about their family goals. Their distinctive reactions created more distance between them. They had difficulty understanding one another and feared disparity about their family-related goals. Their differences, however, were related more to gender-specific reactions about the infertility than to goals about family.

Even though men often react differently, their feelings are equally intense. Men label their feelings differently. They report disappointment but not devastation, even when the infertility appears to be related to male factor causes (Newton & Houle, 1993). They may perceive the infertility as merely a bad break, while their wives report feeling devastated. "I can't believe, sometimes, that Jeremy is even upset," cried Emily during one session. "He just says, 'What is there to talk about?' when I need to feel connected and comforted."

Emily was referencing the different ways they had learned to deal with the pain. Although the infertility may be more painful for women because their identity feels at stake and because they experience monthly physical reminders, the infertility problem can become more isolating for men because they have difficulty discussing such intimate problems. Both spouses experience extensive pain. "While the experience of infertility might be quite different for men and women, distress levels may be quite comparable" (Berg et al., 1991, p. 1077). Although it may appear as though men are not interested in discussing the issues, in fact they may be underreporting their emotional distress because they are less comfortable or able to self-disclose or because they wish to respond in what they believe to be a more socially desirable manner.

RESPONSE TO A DIAGNOSIS OF MALE FACTOR INFERTILITY

The diagnosis of male factor infertility is not talked about as much as the female diagnosis. Men seldom question their own fertility and are therefore unprepared for a male factor diagnosis or their reactions, which are similar to those of women confronted with an infertility diagnosis (Newton & Houle, 1993). Male factor infertility is surrounded with more secrecy than female factor. This is of course related to the cultural stigma surrounding male infertility. "The public view is that 'real men' are strong, virile, and fertile" (Cooper & Glazer, 1994, p. 13).

If the husband is the dominant partner in the marital system, identification as the partner with the infertility problem is especially stressful. Even the most liberated men experience shame and humiliation. These men, like many women, begin to feel their self-esteem plummet as they experience an increased sense of personal failure; they may feel they are being punished for past mistakes or transgressions. Understandably, they begin to question their adequacy as men. Some become impotent or exhibit other sexual problems. For other men, sexual prowess may become more important than their ability to procreate in an attempt to compensate for their perceived inadequacy. "Coitus where there is no possibility of implantation of sperm may be viewed with less worth and is sometimes portrayed as shooting blanks" (Berg et al., 1991, p. 1071).

Many men view fertility more as an issue of virility or masculinity than an issue related to parenting. The powerlessness encountered by infertile men often makes them feel helpless and ineffectual in other parts of their lives. Morris, a successful business owner, talked about his feelings of inadequacy and failure: "I feel so helpless, so much turmoil, so inept. I feel like my masculinity is threatened because I can't get my wife pregnant. I feel bad about not being able to have a child, but my very essence has been attacked too. I don't feel very smart or effective in my office either. I know it's probably related to not being able to concentrate, but I feel inept. And my tennis game has gone downhill. I've lost most of my games this month. I feel powerless and impotent even on the tennis court." Morris is fairly typical of most men who identify first a loss of potency and then the loss of having the biological child, whereas women mourn the loss of the ability to have a child as well as the pregnancy and birth experiences (Newton & Houle, 1993).

Despite the male factor diagnosis, there is a greater involvement of the female in the treatment process, which causes many men to feel excluded (Berg et al., 1991). Even in cases where the husband is being treated with hormones, most often the wife is simultaneously being treated so that she will produce an ample number of satisfactory eggs to be fertilized. This process involves not only daily injections for the wife, but also frequent monitoring of hormone levels and ultrasound examinations in order to monitor the number and size of the eggs. Therefore, the wife is being watched as closely or more closely than the husband and is in frequent interaction with the medical staff. She becomes more familiar with the routines and the staff, which contributes to the husband's feeling like an outsider.

RESOLUTION

Men who cope with infertility through self-centered activities are likely to end up divorced and childless. For Jeremy, the successful professor, staying married and continuing the infertility roller coaster was a choice that was too costly. As they began to discuss separation and eventual divorce, he said, "I love Emily and our life together was great, but I can't take anymore. I like to travel, I like my golf. I'm not willing to be tied to the doctor's office anymore and then maybe tied to a whining child. If that means I have to go it alone, I'll suffer with that at this point in my life." Jason's plan for a resolution to the struggle was to accept infertility and continue life with his wife, Lisa. "I feel just as devastated as Lisa," Jason explained one day. "I resent that we aren't easily fulfilling our dream to create the family we want. I hate not being successful at something. It makes me doubt myself too. I just feel that we have to focus on other parts of our lives."

Factors Contributing to Gender Differences

Although men and women experience many of the same feelings regarding their infertility, they manifest these feelings differently. This often leads to the conclusion that they indeed have very different experiences. Factors such as socialization, how women and men interpret the medical and psychological experience of infertility, their body awareness, and how and to whom they are communicating all contribute to their disparate views.

Socialization

Although it is most likely that men and women have similar feelings and are affected in similar ways by their infertility, there are societal constraints and messages that direct how they will deal with these feelings. The socialization process promotes different meanings in the role that procreation holds for men and women. As discussed earlier, the pregnancy, birth experience, and the fulfillment of the role of mother are important aspects of women's gender identification. "For many women, a pregnant belly is the ultimate sign of femininity; its absence may be interpreted as meaning they are not real women" (Cooper & Glazer, 1994, p. 7). Since people typically assume an inability to procreate is related to female factors, this adds to the social stigma women experience when childless.

Regardless of the extent a woman develops a professional identity, often the picture of herself as a mother remains the psychological backdrop from which she operates. Infertile women often talk about how encounters with groups of mothers make them feel isolated, like second-class citizens, unable to contribute or participate in the "in-group." As as result of this sense of living on the periphery, they need more emotional support than their husbands. Also, these women often engage in more problem-solving and escape coping than their husbands. They are able to find temporary substitutes for the void they feel around mothering by finding other life pursuits that may absorb them for an interim period. For a short time, these diversions are adaptive ways to cope with their emptiness. For example, they take breaks from treatment to finish a college degree, to comply with insurance requirements, or just to reclaim their bodies for a time (Abbey et al., 1991; Sandelowski, 1987). They find ways to regain perspective and to replenish.

Although to Jason, Lisa's husband, Lisa seemed depressed and consumed with her body's nuances, she in fact had mustered some of her resources in a manner that contributed to her well-being: She learned to reach out to other couples rather than isolating. Such connection helped her to feel some support and made her feel less aberrant. According to Newton and Houle (1993), women who accept a great deal of responsibility and who also react with avoidant social behavior rather then engaging social behavior become more vulnerable. So, in fact, her natural tendency to engage with other couples served her well.

Since men are usually more socialized to emphasize the masculinity or virility aspects of procreation rather than the actual parenting aspects, they are less likely to experience gender or role failure issues. A man's identity is not bound to fathering. Although their social interactions may include references to becoming a father, or even discussions about their wife's pregnancy or experience in labor, most men do not mature with a determination to create a family.

Interpreting Medical and Psychological Experiences

Men and women interpret their experiences through lenses they developed in their family and cultural socialization processes. Women are more likely to internalize the infertility experience and blame themselves. "I kept questioning the nurses and the doctors over and over," Gretchen said during one teary session. "I just wanted some answers, a reason why none of these complicated medical things were working. I wanted to know what they *really* thought was wrong with me."

Men are more likely to compartmentalize the situation and to react in a logical manner. Leonard, a 37-year-old car salesman explained: "I don't really care what the reasons are. I know we are having trouble getting pregnant. I also know that we are doing everthing we know to do. But I think we have to discuss moving on soon. All of these doctor visits and talk about doctor visits is interfering with our lives and our marriage." Leonard was more focused on finding a solution than on interpreting his psychological or medical experience.

Men are also more apt to look outside themselves for a rationale. They may blame stress—or even the medical team for not being competent enough. Men can more easily look outside themselves because, as mentioned previously, often their wives and the medical team protect them by inhibiting discussion or the couple may collude with the medical team to maintain secrecy about the infertility itself or the issue of male factor responsibility.

Body Awareness

Although, culturally, both men and women care about their bodies and how they look, women have long felt pressure to remain thin or have a certain figure in order to be desirable. Similarly, women feel pressure to become pregnant in order to fully be a woman. Physiologically, men's and women's bodies experience very different things day to day and month to month. Women have learned to be aware of the nuances of their bodies. For example, prior to monthly menstruation, they are conscious of water retention, irritability, or extreme tiredness; some women claim to be aware of when they are ovulating. Since women's bodies are so regularly tuned to child-bearing processes, women are generally quite sensitized to their bodies and may thus exhibit more distressed responses to the infertility as they regularly face their monthly cycle.

Communication

Since women are more likely to seek confiding relationships and to discuss their infertility, including their feelings about it, they are more likely to receive support or comfort. Likewise, if they continuously discuss infertility-related issues, they are constantly in touch with those issues and their feelings may be consuming or magnified. Since men are apt to partition their feelings and to confide less, they are more able to distance from the infertility and their feelings about the issues. They may, therefore, continue to view the infertility as a part of their functioning but not as a problem that frequently consumes them.

Effect of Gender Differences on the Marital System

Men and women facing infertility do not differ in their appraisals of their overall distress or marital distress. In the initial stages of infertility, both report similar, slightly declining levels of marital and sexual satisfaction (Newton & Houle, 1993). There may be subtle or unconscious adaptations to one another that serve to balance the marital system. Stanton and colleagues (1991) report that husbands indicate less distress as their wives experience greater difficulties from the infertility. Infertile wives score higher on psychosocial distress measures than their husbands and feel more disruption and stress in their personal, social, and sex lives (Wright, Allard, Lecours, & Sabourin, 1989).

As with all experiences of adversity, it appears that many couples come to view infertility difficulties as an impetus for growth, both individually and within the marital system. It is also probable that as treatment continues the partners steel themselves more against the pain and the possibilities of failure. Interestingly, in the middle and later stages of treatment, both men and women reported satisfaction with their marital adjustment, sexual relationship, and degree of communication (Berg et al., 1991; Newton & Houle, 1993). The reality is that in these later stages, to varying degrees, the partners became numb or develop denial about their feelings. "There are just so many fronts I can fight on," explained Gretchen one day in the midst of a fight. "I can't have the students and the superintendent and my husband all bugging me at once. I have less reserves now to fall back on. It seems that every month gets harder." Through the denial or a reframing of the reality, they deceive themselves by creating a new, more palatable reality.

Most aspects of intimacy are hampered by the infertility experience. Lovemaking becomes sex for procreation—and it becomes sex on demand. The sexual and emotional closeness the couple shared in the bedroom now has an almost aversive aspect. "I'm fearful of even asking for lovemaking," explained Jeremy, "because I'm afraid Emily will stop and count what day of month it is or just start crying."

Communication is hampered because it often becomes a discussion of the next medical procedure or how to coordinate the next doctor visit or treatment regimen. Their innermost thoughts are often related to the infertility. As previously discussed, women are more likely to seek social supports to discuss their problems outside the marriage. But if the husband wishes to keep the infertility more private, the wife is then left with few social and emotional supports. According to McEwan and colleagues (1987), women who had a confiding relationship with their spouse showed better adjustment in other areas of their lives. If they do not also confide with friends, however, they lose an important source of support. When the marital partner is the primary confidante, an enormous burden is placed on the marital relationship.

Men have more difficulty in the more general aspects of their marital life (Abbey et al., 1991). They report feelings of loss of control, more interpersonal conflict, and decreased ambition to take on tasks or perform usual routine tasks at home. Marital tension is increased if the spouses fail to recognize one another's struggle and their different coping styles.

Communication breakdowns can occur when the wife wishes to discuss alternatives to biological children or if the husband is unwilling to view infertility as a shared problem to be jointly discussed. Men may often be more optimistic about a pregnancy and therefore less willing to communicate about the infertility because they see it as belaboring the point. "Whatever will happen will happen," Jeremy would often say. "I just don't see any point in going over and over the same 'what if' questions. It's all just conjecture now."

Additionally, because the couple is engaging in so many complex procedures, men are more apt to believe that pregnancy is surely just around the corner. They are not ready or perhaps not willing to consider the alternatives to biological children (Cooper & Glazer, 1994). They are also, as previously discussed, fearful of their wife's physical and emotional pain if they continue treatments. This contributes to their sense of helplessness and inadequacy: They are unable to fix the pain.

For many men, the option of childlessness or child-free living becomes more positive than the continued monthly tension related to treatments, the waiting, the expense, and the ups and downs of surrogacy or adoption. Acceptance of childlessness is associated with increased marital adjustment in men but greater distress in women (Burns, 1993). In fact, infertile couples are more frequently divorced if the husband wants a child and the wife does not. They are more likely to stay married and childless if the wife wants a child, but the husband does not (McDaniel et al., 1992). A husband and wife's different socialization experiences, their different ways of coping with problems, and their individual responses to infertility all play a part in how a couple will ultimately resolve their infertility crisis.

Implications for Therapy

Psychological intervention needs to target both the husband and the wife since adjustment within the marital relationship is a key factor in the ability of these individuals to successfully weather the infertility crisis. Women whose husbands do not participate in the therapy or communicate with them experience more depression as well as marital dissatisfaction (Newton & Houle, 1993). Therapy should focus on strengthening communication while addressing gender differences.

1. The therapist should help the couple understand clearly that men and women differ in their experience of the infertility. As the spouses understand this, their stress levels decrease. Such understanding may also enhance medical compliance (Newton & Houle, 1993).
2. The therapist should also normalize gender differences and discuss their conflict as a male-female experience; spouses become less angry and are able to stop blaming one another when they realize such differences are part of most couples' experiences.
3. The therapist must elicit feelings from both partners and insist that both take responsibility for sharing their inner pain and doubts; if only the wife assumes the emotional responsibility for the infertility, the husband's ability to recognize and resolve his own feelings may be hindered (Burns, 1990).
4. Helping the spouses understand how their different life experiences or contexts contribute to infertility distress relieves much of their tension. Their awareness of the factors that contribute to gender differences and how they affect one another helps them tolerate their partner's distinct reactions.

Once the partners realize that different aspects of the situation may be more stressful for one than the other, and that each adapts to stress differently, they are ready to learn how to minimize their distress (Berg et al., 1991). Merely explaining and discussing their distress often serves only to increase their unhappiness. Following is a list of techniques that will help the partners minimize their distress, and thus relieve their frustration.

1. Suggest they limit the amount of time they spend discussing infertility issues.

2. Direct the husband to merely listen to his wife when she talks about her feelings; he need not try to fix the problem. For example, in order to cope with her depression, the wife will need to be able to discuss her issues around self-blame. Having her husband respond and explain his own feelings, including a lack of blame, will help them bond and begin to restructure their relationship.

3. Teach the couple communication skills that counter gender differences in communication styles; this will help them hear and understand one another more clearly.

4. Because men concentrate more on their wife's pain, encourage the husband to accept his own pain, particularly his sense of loss. Like their wives, men experience the fear of not achieving pregnancy and thus the potential loss of a biological child. They also feel a loss of control that comes from being at the mercy of numerous tests and procedures and, as previously mentioned, from their inability to fix the situation for their wives. Oftentimes they feel they have lost their companion as well as their lover.

5. Explain certain gender-specific coping strategies. For example, when men try to fix the situation by becoming less expressive than their wives or becoming stoic, their wives interpret these behaviors as ignoring or withdrawing behaviors. Similarly, if the husband tries to fix the situation by calling an adoption agency or another such intervention activity, his wife may interpret this as failure on her part to provide him with something very critical, or she may feel pressure to hurry and get pregnant. When the therapist explains that these behaviors relate to his inability to fix her pain, she can hear it as a more caring response.

6. Encourage the spouses to discuss their motives, differences, and goals; sometimes writing their thoughts and feelings in letters to each other or in an open journal is a less threatening way of communicating this information.

7. Help the partners negotiate a time limit around their medical treatments; this can provide a forum to discuss their goals, as well as the numerous options for family building if that's what they wish to pursue. The husband may be more willing than the wife to pursue other roles as a substi-

tute for parenting. This needs to be accepted and encouraged while the woman's need to express her parenting needs is recognized and validated.

As each partner begins to communicate his or her fears and sense of inadequacy, the spouses free themselves from many misconceptions and pave the way for increasing their intimacy. They lean more on one another rather than fearing the other as a critic or feeling they are a disappointment to their partner. They can begin the tasks of rebuilding their individual and couple self-images. They can again begin to rely on their own inner strength and the strong inner core of the couple system, which they had previously trusted and from which they originally drew strength.

5

STRUGGLING WITH INFERTILITY: THE CONTEXT OF RELIGIOUS AND CULTURAL PARADIGMS

PARENTHOOD, FAMILY, AND FERTILITY connote different things in different cultures. The degree of importance of these issues and the different meanings attributed to them can become a source of comfort, pain, or conflict between marital partners. In all cultures, young adulthood represents a time of enormous psychological, financial, and physical growth. It is a time when young people are expected to make their own way in the world. They leave the comforts of home, whether that means leaving the warm family hearth or the safe routines of college life. It is during this time that many individuals form lasting relationships that become the basis for the formation of their own nuclear family. According to Erikson (1950), this is a time of generativity or, as Freud postulated, a time when parenthood becomes a normal outcome of the development to adulthood.

It is indeed truly challenging for two people coming from different families, different cultures, who have not lived in the same places and who do not share the symbols of nationality, religion, race, class, or gender, to forge a relationship—much less navigate the rocky seas of infertility. "Being human is an endless effort to collect our distributed selves from all the locations where they are scattered, forging them into a more coherent account of who we are" (DiNicola, 1997, p. 14).

When Jim and Maria called for therapy, they identified their presenting symptoms as poor communication and a sense of enormous distance between them. They did not yet understand that their issues related to attempts to integrate their "scattered selves" as individuals, as well as establish their couple system. Maria came from a traditional Puerto Rican family, close-knit and in constant intimate communication. Jim's family, in contrast, was an English and Irish mix, more distant, private, and comfortable with minimal communication. It became clear in the process of their therapy that the strain they were experiencing was due to their infertility. This was exacerbated by their inability to bridge their cultural differences. "He just takes everything in stride," Maria complained one session. "Another month goes by without a pregnancy and he doesn't blink an eye. Doesn't seem to phase him. If our house would burn down I swear he would just stand there and shrug his shoulders. He doesn't react to so many important things. My family can't understand him either."

Erikson (1950) defines identity as a process connected to the core of the individual. This core is also made up of one's communal culture. Therefore, if there are cultural mandates regarding procreation, infertile individuals experience a great deal of internal and external conflict vis-à-vis their cultural prescriptives. In most Western cultures, until the early to mid-twentieth century, the sole role of married women was childbearing and rearing. Since women had limited access to birth control or abortion and limited political impact, they were relegated to follow historical precedents in terms of their role definitions.

Individuals from different cultural or socioeconomic backgrounds suffering with infertility share similar psychological and emotional issues; however, the degree and severity of each person's experience will differ (Baluch, Al-Shawaf, & Craft, 1992). One's individual identity as well as the communal identity is at stake. The religious or cultural diversity of the couple system thus creates a powerful context for the couple to navigate as they move through life.

Different Religious Perspectives

Religious differences can be a divisive force in a couple's marriage, tearing the fabric of the couple's carefully woven life tapestry. This is particularly true when there are unanticipated crises such as infertility. Religious influence over fertility and infertility can be significant. The Catholic, Jewish, and Mormon religions, for example, teach that a woman's primary role and significance lies with her ability to create new life. It follows, therefore, that when a woman is confronted with infertility, she questions her worth. If she is childless, she is useless. Early religious writings used the term "barren" and allowed annulment of the marriage when a wife was infertile (Salzer, 1991), although not if the husband was infertile (Eck Menning, 1988).

Couples often feel pressure from their religious codes as well as directly from clergy. "I remember the priest talking to us before we were married," Jim explained one session. "He was clear about our responsibility to continue our heritage, to have children, and of course to bring them up in the Catholic tradition." Maria added, "You know, the priests don't talk to young couples much about sex anymore these days, but our priest was clear that there are those moral issues about sex. He emphasized that sex should create pregnancies and babies. It brings back all those messages from my childhood that sex was sinful unless it was to make babies. If you can't do that, you feel so inadequate and helpless."

The Old Testament discusses fertility and worthiness. Women who found favor with the Lord ultimately conceived. Five famous women—Sarah, Rachel, Leah, Hannah, and Elizabeth—not only conceived, but did so repeatedly even at what was reported to be an advanced age. As a consequence of this connection between fertility and a woman's value or favor with the Lord, infertility is seen as punishment, signaling that she is out of favor with God. Often, when couples feel guilty about past behaviors, such as premarital sex or adolescent rebelliousness, they will attribute the difficulties to punishment from God. Brigette, a successful hospital administrator, explained one day, "My Mom was a very religious person and, I think, often superstitious. She would threaten me when she was angry by telling me God would punish me. Now I feel like she's getting her revenge. I sure can't otherwise explain all of this pain."

Sometimes the message is not so much about sin but about pressure to carry on the religion and religious heritage. For example, Orthodox Judaism teaches that without children the union between two people is unfilled. In fact, infertility becomes conspicuous because it is expected that procreation will follow soon after marriage.

It is understandable that religious pressures experienced by infertile couples can cause them to internalize their condition and attribute it to personal failings. Some couples, as previously mentioned, feel it is a punishment for sins they have committed. Some see it as a form of suffering related to a special message from God, a mystical message that is beyond their ability to comprehend. Others see their infertility as a message from God to push them to rethink their life plans. Jason saw his and Lisa's infertility as a tough hurdle to overcome in order to grow up or learn humility. "We've just been having so much fun," Jason commented one day, "that we thought the most important things in life were our careers, earning big bucks, and having a good time. Our infertility has brought us up short. I think God wanted us to learn some humility and look more seriously at the bigger issues in life."

Many couples experience guilt around their infertility rather than perceiving it as a potential growth experience. "They experience a phase in which they try to atone for transgressions and strike bargains with God. But when all the prayers, penance, and 'good behavior' fail, their rage is likely to intensify" (Salzer, 1991, p. 167). Religion does not teach them about injustice. In fact, this betrayal becomes one of the most devastating experiences they have ever faced. "I thought my divorce was the worst thing I would ever have to face," cried Melissa, a high-powered financial planner. "I felt so let down, so betrayed by this man I thought loved me. But now even God has betrayed me." Ironically, the more religious the person, the greater the intensity of the emphasis on family and children. A Mormon woman receives elaborate instructions on motherhood that affirms the strength of the religious doctrine. A Chassidic woman's identity is incomplete without an association to family and children (Silverstein, 1995). "We really didn't want to consider divorce," explained Sara, an Orthodox Jewish woman. "But I was pretty fearful for a long time that Joshua would abandon me because of our infertility. I don't even want to think about what would have happened to us and our daily lives if we hadn't finally conceived. It took a terrible toll on our marriage. I cried a lot. He prayed a lot with his brothers and father. We could hardly talk at all, just about the mundane daily routine stuff." It is a cruel twist of fate—and a test of their faith—when these couples have to confront infertility. It threatens their place in the community and challenges the very essence of their belief systems.

The Impact of Ethnicity

An individual's ethnic values and identification come down through many generations and serve as strong, stable life forces. "Ethnicity remains a vital force in this country, a major form of group identification, and a major determinant of our family patterns and belief systems" (McGoldrick, Pearce, & Giordano, 1982, p. 3). Since ethnicity plays a significant role throughout the life cycle, partners receive messages that influence the degree of pressure they feel regarding interactions with their families of origin and the pressures to create their own nuclear family.

Although the degree of significance regarding women's roles as fertility symbols varies across cultures, infertility is a crisis in all cultures. This has been true throughout recorded history. The infertility experienced by King Henry VIII of England is a widely known example that revolutionized religious as well as moral systems of an entire country. Even in cases of less known or less influential persons, individual infertility can have an effect on a community and the larger society.

Since one's ethnic identity evokes deep feelings that relate to the continuity of the family over generations and even centuries, when it is not understood or is conflicted the marital system is affected. Since each ethnic group provides its own cultural norms and values, and therefore its own system by which to solve problems, each partner needs to understand the power of those rules in order to bridge the chasm they're experiencing. The solutions, too, will be related to the lenses through which each partner views the situation. If the couple understands how each partner's ethnicity influences his or her reactions as well as proposed solutions, the marital system can transcend the cultural differences more readily. "It isn't that I don't care," Jim explained in a particularly angry therapy session, "I'm in a lot of pain too, Maria. And I do talk with my family about all of this. It's just that they don't react as emotionally as your Mom or your sister. It doesn't mean they don't react. And it doesn't mean they don't care." Jim's explanation provided an important clarification for Maria. It helped her become less angry and resentful, thus providing a bridge for them to talk about and resolve their misunderstandings.

Partners are generally so entrenched in their unique cultural or ethnic roots that they often don't realize how particular their dynamics are to their spouse. They do not realize that making the implicit more explicit will help to demystify the strange or the unknown. Assisting them to specifically label, clarify, and express their identification with these codes or values helps create a perspective for the partner that is less threatening and that can, in fact, become a unifying bond as they work together to find creative ways of accommodating their differences.

Seeking Solutions

Spouses of different cultural backgrounds may encounter adjustment difficulties in the marriage. When differences in gender reactions to life and infertility are added to this mix, the couple has a recipe for stress within the marital system. For example, certain ethnic groups, such as Italians, Greeks, and Jews, more commonly seek high levels of interaction with medical or psychological caregivers. WASP, Irish, and Scandinavian families, on the other hand, are more likely to deal with problems by minimizing or denying the need for help from medical or psychological caregivers (McGoldrick, Preto, Hines, & Lee, 1991). So when an Italian man is married to an Irish woman, they may argue about when to seek medical intervention for childlessness or who will present for infertility treatment. They are also likely to experience frustrations about how and with whom to discuss future treatment options.

Acceptable Solutions

In addition, the choice of acceptable solutions to infertility is also a powerful issue. For example, Puerto Rican families have a deep sense of family commitment, obligation, and responsibility. There are flexible boundaries between families and the surrounding community so that child lending, a practice of allowing a child to spend significant time in households other than her immediate family's, is common and accepted. Thus, Maria felt more comfortable than her husband, Jim, a man from an English and Irish family, when surrounded by children, even though she was experiencing childlessness. She also felt at ease considering adoption if they could not conceive. "We both love kids a lot," Jim said, somewhat defensively. "It's just that Maria can warm up to and love any kid. I can't. I don't know, maybe the chemistry just isn't there or something. So I'm not sure I could love an adopted child who wasn't mine, if you know what I mean. I think I need to see signs that he's like me, or Maria, before I could warm up to him."

Italians, on the other hand, have tight boundaries against outsiders and define themselves first in terms of their family ties. Although this makes it difficult for the infertile couple in terms of identification as a family, it does not preclude adoption. Adoption is an unlikely alternative for a Greek family, whose tight, definitive family boundaries stress blood lines.

The Marital Agreement

In some cultures, the inability to bear a child may represent an incapacity to comply with the original terms of the marital agreement. For example, Iranian males consider children as insurance for future support. Pressure and strong expectations are placed on couples to bear children at an early stage in the marriage. "I knew my parents would try to influence me to leave Sari," explained Sharif one tearful session. "I was afraid to tell them about our infertility. I knew it would mean nothing to them that I really loved her. That doesn't mean much to my family or in my culture if you can't produce a family."

The Significance of Children

Ethnic and cultural groups place varying degrees of emphasis on family and children. Chinese Americans believe the spousal relationship is secondary to the parent-child relationship. In fact, Confucius believed the family constituted the most important institution in society. Many women marry young in order to have many children (McGoldrick, Preto, et al., 1991). Nodal life events—birth, marriage, and death—are significant events in the Chinese family; however, a baby's one-month birthday is a particularly momentous occasion, which becomes a large extended-family affair. African-Americans regard family relationships as important for promoting survival. Like the Chinese, they also place a higher value on the parental role than on the spousal role. Therefore, these couples often wait only a short time after marriage before their first pregnancies. Some young African-American women also choose to have children outside of marriage rather than risk childlessness (McGoldrick, Preto, et al., 1991). Similarly, Puerto Rican women marry young and have many children. "Children are seen as the poor man's wealth, the caretakers of the old and as a symbol of fertility" (McGoldrick, Preto, et al., 1991, p. 554).

When partners represent different cultures and then confront infertility, intense levels of intra- and interpersonal conflict can occur. "She just doesn't understand how much pressure I feel," explained Sharif, tearfully. "In the Iranian culture I feel shamed. I have a beautiful wife, but she is a corporate vice president, not a mother. My family does not understand. They make fun of me. They do not understand infertility. They think she makes all the rules and runs the house and doesn't care about kids. She doesn't feel these pressures. Her family reinforces her career. They tell her she has lots of time to have children."

Jewish families represent a unique set of pressures and expectations, since they constitute both a cultural and religious configuration. The religious precepts place a premium on procreation and the ability to replenish the group. Ethnically, Jewish families place a strong emphasis on the family. The family is the core of religious and cultural traditions and rituals. The Bar or Bat Mitzvah, although centered around a religious occasion representing a child's admission to adulthood in the religious community, has become a cultural event. Other holidays also have a religious backdrop, but have evolved into child-oriented cultural occasions with animated storytelling and grand celebration. The childless Jewish couple thus often confronts occasions that magnify their emptiness. "I just can't bear going to your parents' for Passover," Carol explained to Craig. "All the kids participate in the Seder and then run around looking for their special reward that Grandpa hid. It just emphasizes our own horrible situation. It's never just a holiday, it's always like a mini carnival. We have nothing to contribute."

Gender Roles within the Family

Different cultures also have covert and overt rules governing gender roles. Thus, couples who intermarry experience not only differing pressures regarding family building, but also gender differences regarding involvement with and raising of the children. WASP males are more isolated at home due to cultural values that push them to place career first. As a result, they may feel irrelevant or inadequate in terms of child-rearing. Consequently, it is also unlikely that they will feel much relevance or comfort in dealing with the infertility issues. Similarly, Irish men are peripherally involved in their families, while the women are overly central. Children are not the center of adult attention, yet it is not uncommon for mothers to overindulge and overprotect their sons and expect too much from their daughters (McGoldrick, Preto, et al., 1991). Since the Irish typically are stoic, Irish women would be less likely to communicate their pain about infertility, but perhaps more likely to overcompensate a son who is born after infertility has been experienced.

Puerto Rican fathers are considered the heads of the family but have no child or household responsibilities. Machismo, particularly virility, is assumed and revered. Infertility is particularly threatening to the couple, both in terms of inability to flaunt the male's virility as well as the inability to add to the kinship network.

In a somewhat different variation, Jewish families place a lot of responsibility on both partners to attend to child-rearing, although there is no emphasis on virility and machismo. They typically have more egalitarian relationships, both in terms of decision-making and child-rearing, although they may divide the type of responsibilities.

Class Differences

Differences in socioeconomic class can also contribute to conflict and pressures the couple may experience around the issues of children and family. According to Zoldbrod (1993), class differences affect men's attitudes toward children and family. Women and men in the lower and lower-middle classes express an expected natural progression from marriage to parenthood. Lower-class men believe having children is an unquestioned expectation. In the case of male factor infertility, they deny that it is a threat to their virility; their wives, however, indicate it clearly threatens one of their expected roles as a husband. Men feel guilt and shame that they are letting their wives down.

By comparison, the professional class experiences an intense elongation of the process of forming a family (Fulmer, 1989). Professional couples typically complete graduate degrees before they even consider marriage. When they marry, they struggle to prevent pregnancy for a number of years. "It is so ironic," complained Iris, a 38-year-old engineer, during a therapy session. "Carl always wanted to get settled, buy our house, and pay off our student loans before we had children. All those years he worried about us accidentally becoming pregnant. Now I'm so angry about it. When my parents married they immediately started having their babies. But no, we had to be like his snobby family—to be successful and have some status before we could have our babies." Even though Iris was successful and a highly respected engineer, she still carried her family's lower-middle-class value system, particularly regarding family and children. Initially, she was willing to go along with Carl's upper-middle-class value system, and in fact aspired to those values in many ways. But when she confronted infertility, she came to resent their class differences and the imposition of those values on her childbearing.

Not surprisingly, partners from different socioeconomic backgrounds often experience similar struggles when faced with a crisis. In fact, socioeconomic variables may influence the factors that motivate a couple to seek or not seek infertility treatment. Even when the infertility has been addressed and dealt with through medical channels, the partners are often oriented differently to the emotional impact and how they will deal with that. Children, or a lack of, represent different meanings to a partner from an upper-class background than a partner from a lower-class background. These socioeconomic variables become further complicated by differences in educational background. As David, an auto mechanic, explained during one session, "I knew Ellen shouldn't get her master's degree. She puts so much energy into her career. She kept putting off having our family, and now we have this infertility stuff. I'm not sure she really minds, to tell you the truth. I just wanted us to be a big happy family, to go camping and skiing with our kids like my family did. But she always has one more talk to give or report to write. It seems like she's more interested in her reports than in having kids."

Regardless of whether the differences are religious or socioeconomic, the partners find themselves in uncharted territory without a map. Although family rituals provided some guidance as they were growing up, their current nuclear family structure has not yet formulated a useful roadmap.

Effects of the Cultural and Religious Differences on the Couple System

Cultural messages are powerful and can place tremendous pressure on individuals and therefore on the marital system. "Pressure on couples to bear children comes from a combination of mythology, religion, culture, and society" (Eck Menning, 1988, p. 100). Our cultural backgrounds pattern our thinking, feeling, and behavior. They play a large role in determining how we work or relax, whether or in what ways we celebrate holidays or rituals, and perhaps even what we eat. Under the best of circumstances, couples who intermarry experience major challenges to their relationship when confronted with these differences in the context of their family and cultural value systems. Since intermarriage affects every level of a system, from the individual to the ethnic groups involved to the society (McGoldrick et al., 1991), the problems encountered in the usual marital life transitions can be exacerbated by the distinctive cultural messages each partner carries. Since cultures generally favor motherhood, they may label couples who have delayed childbearing or are silently infertile as "selfish" and "materialistic."

Some cultural or ethnic groups view marriage as a union of two working partners, while others view it as a vehicle for the rearing of children or as an extension of the family network. If a partner dealing with infertility is part of the latter group, he or she experiences a conflict in ethnic identity, which can precipitate the loss of a sense of self. "I feel lots of pressure from my family to have grandkids for my Mom," explained Maria. "And Jim just doesn't understand this. I know he wants kids and his Mom will tease every once in a while, but he doesn't feel it as a pressure. Maybe because he's a guy or just from a different family, but it doesn't affect how he feels about himself or his life. It makes me wonder if there's something wrong with me or with our marriage that he's not more upset about all of this."

Since many attitudes about fertility and infertility have remained in the realm of myths, taboos, and superstitions, couples feel betrayed by their religious teachings. They were taught that if they followed the Golden Rule, believed in God, and were decent people, they would reap the rewards of a good life. Instead, what these couples experience is a lack of desired rewards with no reasonable explanation for their plight. Instead of the support they seek from their culture and religion, they feel pressure imposed on them. These couples may retreat from their religion when going through infertility.

Similarly, stress from the couple's diverse ethnic backgrounds compounds the stress of life-cycle transitions, since "ethnicity interacts with the family life cycle at every stage" (McGoldrick et al., 1982, p. 17). Couples who are stopped short at the generative stage of the life cycle experience severe emotional conflict. They are unable to transition through the usual family experiences or family rituals. "Since life-cycle rituals enable us to begin to rework our sense of self and our relationships as required by life's changes, the lack of such rituals can make change more difficult" (Imber-Black & Roberts, 1992, p. 283). Partners experience internal dissonance and interpersonal tension. They fight about holidays with family, about how or whether to celebrate holidays in their own household. It is understandable that they also fight about their own disappointment and emptiness. They had anticipated creating their own rituals as well as sharing traditional ones with their families. However, for these couples, the familiar comfort that rituals create is glaringly absent. Sometimes they do not create or participate in rituals because they wish to avoid any reminders of their infertility or questions from others about a stressful life-cycle event such as a miscarriage or stillbirth. Normal conflicts set off by a couple's intermarriage, whether inter-ethnic or inter-religious, become aggravated by life-cycle stresses. The families of origin may conflict to the point of precipitating a cutoff. The couple may already have become excluded from family rituals prior to their infertility, but the resulting isolation and pain related to the infertility exacerbate the cutoff and thus the couple's stress.

Implications for Therapy

Address the Partners' Pain

Initially, therapy needs to transcend the cultural, ethnic, or religious issues in order to address the partners' pain. "A family therapist joins these strangers in search of the familiar and the reassuring" (DiNicola, 1997, p. 32). Once the therapist meets the spouses across cultures, she must facilitate the cultural translation of their distress. The meaning of their anguish must become more accessible and understandable not only to the therapist but also to the partners. The therapist must push them to specifically describe their inner experiences, feelings, and thoughts. Then the therapy can progress to deal with the larger sytemic issues, which include both the marital system and the families-of-origin contexts, that is, their cultural, ethnic, and religious backgrounds.

As ethnic groups differ in their experience of pain and how they communicate about pain, there may be increased distress for the inter-ethnic couple. One partner may experience a level of pain that the other cannot comprehend because of their different backgrounds. "If only he would talk to me," cried Maria during an emotional session. "I just feel so lonely, so abandoned. Everyone in my family is screaming and crying, and Jim just does nothing."

Therapist: Maria, I can understand how lonely you must feel. What also impresses me, however, is the extent of Jim's pain, although I know it is hard for you to see it. His Irish and English parents just do not outwardly express their emotional pain. Jim is more used to that way of dealing with pain. Your family, from the Puerto Rican culture, has a different, more emotional way of approaching such problems.

Jim: Yeah, and Maria, you know how much I love you and your family. It's still foreign to me, to be so emotional about life, and it makes me uncomfortable.

Therapist: Whoops. I don't think you meant to sound judgmental there, Jim. I think the emphasis should be on your *different* ways of handling things rather then on the positive or negative.

Jim: Absolutely. I admire and like the way you deal with us, Maria. I wish I could sometimes be more emotional, and I do try, believe it or not. Please understand that I'm in there pitching even though I'm not effusive about it.

Couples need assistance in negotiating such differences between their cultural contexts. Each partner must explore the possibility that the spouse's culture is in some way threatening. What might be discovered is that a partner is afraid of losing her own cultural identity or that she feels disloyal when adopting observances from a foreign culture. Beneath the anger, there may be a fear of losing roots. All of these issues must be presented in the therapy and thoroughly discussed or confronted by both partners. Otherwise, such underlying fears will add unnecessary and crippling stress to a predicament already fraught with anxiety (DiNicola, 1997).

"Typically we tolerate differences better when we are not under stress, and indeed find them appealing. When stress is added to a system, our tolerance for difference diminishes, and we become frustrated if we are not understood in ways that fit our wishes and expectations" (McGoldrick et al., 1991, p. 574). Therefore, it is important for the partners to reach an understanding of the meaning of infertility to each of them. The couple needs assistance in negotiating the differences in their cultural contexts; to "build a bridge between what is genuinely our own and other strange experiences" (DiNicola, 1997, p. 117). Even though their tendency is to become angry over the misunderstandings, the partners can learn to perceive their diverseness in a different context, allowing them to relate in more constructive ways. When struggling through such conflict, they glean an increased appreciation for their differences and subsequently enjoy an increased sense of intimacy.

Discuss Faith and Support

The infertility crisis often acts as a catalyst in an individual's or couple's spiritual life. Thus, another goal of the therapy is to help infertile couples find comfort through an exploration of their spirituality. Formalized religion can help some couples ascribe meaning to conditions beyond their control. Developmentally, individuals experience many changes in their need for religion. For example, people commonly turn away from their religion or ethnic or cultural heritage during the turbulent adolescent years but return when they marry or create their own nuclear families.

If religion was once a source of support, it is often helpful to encourage an embittered infertile couple to return to their faith. Remind the couple that religion "has comforted people in times of tragedy and offered principles by which to live, providing a system of values and sense of direction, especially during times of crisis" (Salzer, 1991, p. 160). The values that their religion previously provided can become a comfort once again. Religion can also provide solace and furnish answers to complex human questions and dilemmas. Their faith may give them a sense of direction when they feel they are flailing from the shock and betrayal of infertility.

Many individuals find that a return to their religion may offer a chance to relieve some of their guilt over past behaviors. They may feel a sense of "cleansing" from a confession of these real or imagined sins. This sense of cleansing or being forgiven is a great benefit in helping them accept and resolve their infertility.

While some turn to religion in times of crisis, others turn away at that moment because they feel betrayed by God. Those who find little or no comfort in religion must be helped to find alternative sources of support. Meditation and yoga may provide peace and a form of spiritual uplifting for some. Others must seek support from understanding family members, from other couples who are struggling with infertility, or from support groups available through therapists or RESOLVE (see chapter 3 for a more detailed discussion of these support options).

Create Rituals to Bridge Cultural Differences

In our culture at large, there are no familiar and accepted rituals for many crucial life-cycle transitions, such as leaving home or divorce. Likewise, critical life crises such as pregnancy loss or early menopause occur with little acknowledgment or support from the larger culture despite far-reaching reverberations for the individuals and the couple system. So the couple needs assistance to create their own innovative rituals. A therapist can help a couple examine the meanings of their individual experience and the impact of the medical diagnosis of infertility. It is useful for each partner to draw on cultural traditions used in their own family of origin. "The symbols and actions available in cultural material and family traditions can be drawn upon and [reclaimed and recreated] in ways that fit new contexts and altered meanings" (Laird, 1988, p. 357).

Whether the couple has experienced a loss through infertility or a pregnancy loss, or a positive addition such as an adoption, they need to create a melding of their heritages in order to establish ways to commemorate these significant life events. Creating their own rituals becomes therapeutic because it serves to help them begin to heal and simultaneously helps them become more bonded. "After our miscarriage, we were just at such odds. We found it hard to talk about, until Ken came up with the idea of creating a ritual as a way to let it go," explained Stephanie. "We used my idea of Ken and I reading some poetry and some words from a few of the prophets, followed by a gathering of friends. We created something like a wake, a happy occasion similar to what we did with his family after his uncle died. It really helped us move from the somber, sad stuff, back into a celebration of life. It helped me see the strengths in his family's way of doing things too." "We had a naming ceremony for our son in our synagogue," Craig said, when he called to tell me of their adoption. "It was a wonderful integration of our families and our cultures. We structured it so that it had portions similar to a baptism for Carol's family and other portions referencing Jewish themes and symbols. It was so healing for Carol and me and wonderful for our families as well." "Therapeutic rituals yield dramatic shifts in the areas of membership and beliefs by balancing the themes of similarities and differences" (Whiting, 1988, p. 227).

As spouses sort through what is meaningful and as they communicate about these powerful, often comforting images, they create a common focus, an integration of their differences. Thus, the couple system can learn to draw strength from their differences.

More importantly, the partners become more united through the process of establishing their own unique rituals, a meaningful sequence which they understand and share. Since families crave continuity, successful therapy will include giving a couple the tools to blend their own traditions such that each partner feels that continuity between family of origin and their own nuclear family has been achieved. Since "we move from the familiar to the strange, seeking to familiarize even the most foreign experience" (DiNicola, 1997, p. 28), the therapist's ultimate task is to help the couple build bridges between the individuals' notions of family and their particular cultural heritages, to weave their differences into a meaningful and intimate tapestry.

6

WHEN INFERTILITY IS NOT THE PRESENTING COMPLAINT: USING GENOGRAMS TO EXPLORE THE ISSUES

WHEN JACK AND DARLEEN explained their reasons for seeking therapy, they didn't imagine that the core issues related to their infertility. "He doesn't listen to me," complained Darleen, a 38-year-old architect. "He's always so preoccupied. When he does respond, he's critical and impatient." Jack, a 40-year-old human resources executive for a large corporation, was quite accustomed to defending himself, "Well, you are always so worried about every little thing. You don't set priorities, so I can't tell what's really important and what I can ignore. You could be taking care of more of these issues yourself."

Both expressed feeling as if they were constantly in crisis. They found it difficult to discern a significant issue from a relatively simple one. Decisions often felt complicated and burdensome. The therapist asked, "How long have you felt this way? Did you feel these things before your 3-year-old son was born?" They believed so. In fact, upon further exploration they realized that many of these feelings surfaced and became exacerbated when they were going through infertility medical procedures; they were able to recall the anxiety, their preoccupation with Darlene's body and her cycles, and their feelings of helplessness and being out of control. When they ultimately became pregnant, they never thought they needed to sort out the previous dark months and years—they were having too much fun focusing on the arrival of the baby.

This is typical of many couples who have experienced infertility. These couples will enter therapy with various complaints but not necessarily perceive the pain they are experiencing as related to their past bouts with infertility. They do not perceive infertility as an ongoing issue. Many feel that by achieving parenthood or a child-free resolution they have resolved their infertility. But like any crisis, it is never erased or eradicated from their life experiences, attitudes, or reactions.

Although almost all couples encounter difficulties and obstacles in their lives together, infertility represents an impediment that is different from other hurdles couples may confront. This is particularly true for couples who have achieved parenthood. Since approximately 95 percent of newly married couples want and expect to have biological children of their own at some point in their lives (Matthews & Matthews, 1986), it makes sense that difficulty becoming pregnant will present a severe blow to a couple's goals and their ongoing functioning. Because most couples attempt to keep it private, it is difficult to realize the extent of residual pain, anxiety, or depression that may be attributable to those distressful times. Additionally, since most couples carefully choose when and with whom to disclose their problems with fertility, they are often alone with their pain and dependent on one another for support and solace. The isolation adds to the burden on the marital system, creating increased stress for the partners.

Burns (1990) reported that 76 percent of respondents in her study believed infertility had caused conflict in their marriage; this group reported a significantly higher incidence of marital problems than the control group. Marital problems included disruption in sexual relations and disagreements about further medical treatment or adoption. The new ART procedures are so stressful to couples that many feel somatic and psychological symptoms, such as depression and anxiety, following failure of one of these procedures (Baram, Tourtelot, Muechler, & Huang, 1988). Burns (1990) found that 85 percent of the partners in her study rated infertility as a negative experience that created disruption in their lives combined with feelings of anger, hopelessness, frustration, and a sense of being overwhelmed. "I try to remain 'up' for Sally," explained

Peter, a 42-year-old computer analyst, "so I just ignore my own sadness. I try to deal with it through my athletics and just tell myself I have to make the best of it." Most couples also reported communication problems during their trials with infertility. In addition to disagreements about the actual treatments, they felt their spouse failed to understand or acknowledge their perspective. Often one partner had a greater investment in the treatment or the outcome, which aggravated the communication problems, the sense of conflict, and the distance between them. The marriage frequently became secondary to one partner's needs and desires for a child.

It is important that the therapist be aware of the effects of infertility and know how to pose significant questions in order to sift out information about infertility. Information about previous infertility and its impact can become evident during the assessment phase of therapy. Family of origin issues as well as the couple's historical development can yield information about planned or unplanned pregnancies, infertility, abortions, or adoptions. The genogram can be a valuable tool for assisting the couple or family in identifying residual infertility-related issues.

Using Genograms to Discover Unresolved Infertility Issues

Sam and Alexandra called to schedule marital therapy after a particularly destructive fight. "We've been having many of these fights lately," Sam explained. "Alex is just not the same since her dad died. She seems to fly off the handle at anything." Sam and Alexandra had been married for 18 years. Alexandra, at 41, was a hard-driving financial planner who had just gone out on her own. Sam, at 46, had just become a partner in an accounting firm. They both enjoyed success, respect, and financial rewards in their careers. They loved to travel, dress well, eat at expensive restaurants, and go to exotic places for long weekends.

"Everyone thinks we have the most romantic, exciting life," Alexandra sighed during one session, "and it did seem great for a long time. But I guess when my dad was sick I just started questioning all of this. I'm not sure where the meaning is anymore. It just doesn't seem like our lifestyle offers any meaning. Sam works and then comes home and works. During the tax season I hardly even see him. He's a stranger and doesn't have much to say when he is there."

It wasn't until Alex and Sam began giving the information to complete their genogram that it became apparent that they had gone through a period of infertility and in fact had not worked to resolve those scars. They had ultimately just let the ball drop and had not made a deliberate decision about children in their lives.

Often, as in the case of Jack and Darleen or Sam and Alexandra, the individuals are not aware that the pain they are experiencing is related to the past trauma of the infertility roller coaster. They do not realize the reverberations that infertility continues to send through their couple or family system. The genogram provides a format to gain the insights into the powerful residue left by this crisis and to finally put it into a perspective.

There are certain behaviors that are common to couples who have experienced a crisis of any kind, who have struggled for a long time with factors beyond their control. Such behaviors include anxious behaviors, such as excessive worry, feelings of doom or hopelessness, or hypervigilance. If they have been told by a teacher, relative, or therapist that they are overprotective, they do not connect such behaviors with their arduously attained parenthood. They do not connect their negative doomsday reactions to life's occurrences with the series of monthly "failures" they experienced. It is often a relief to these families and couples to be able to discover the connections. When they see the larger picture indicated by the genogram, they feel less guilt and more control and power over their lives, their marriage, and their family.

Exploring the family history, births, and deaths is a fairly common practice among family therapists. The infertility specialist, however, must also ask more specific questions pertinent to the couple's family-building. For example: Did the spouses *choose* to postpone having children? Did they deliberately decide not to have children at all? Were the long gaps between children intentional or the result of other factors, such as secondary infertility, a miscarriage, or marital discord? An initial assessment may produce a genogram similar to the first one depicted in figure 6.1. Upon further, very focused questioning, an additional layer of their relationship is uncovered. The hovering cloud of infertility is unveiled and can thus be addressed and diffused.

The absence of children may reflect a mutual decision to be child-free, to postpone having children, mutual ambivalence, disagreement, or infertility/subfertility.

Couples experiencing primary infertility (no children) as a result of chronic miscarriage may not volunteer the information when asked about children or deaths in the family.

Secondary infertility (have one or more children but want another) is just as stressful as primary infertility.

Long gaps between children may reflect mutual choice, unintentional pregnancy, a period of disagreement, or a period of infertility.

Long periods of marriage prior to having children may reflect mutual choice, disagreement about timing, or infertility. Issues of infertility may not be volunteered even if they are in the couple's awareness. Long-awaited children or children following a miscarriage or stillbirth may be favored or highly protected.

Most couples adopt only after efforts for a biological child have failed. While most volunteer that the child is adopted, they may not volunteer any unresolved issues of infertility, misgivings about adoption, or fear of birth-mother contact.

While infertile couples who have adopted are no more likely to later have a biological child than those who don't adopt (occurs in only about 5 percent of cases), any preferential feelings for the biological child may produce guilt or denial and influence parenting behaviors.

Single individuals may or may not be single by choice. Those who are fertile may be more distressed by the lack of a child then lack of a spouse.

Gay and lesbian couples may want a child but perceive or experience unequal access to adoption, surrogacy, or donor options.

Many believe their desire for children will be satisfied by marrying a spouse who has sole or joint custody of chidren by a previous marriage. When these hopes are dashed, they encounter a form of involuntary childlessness, which is just as painful as infertility.

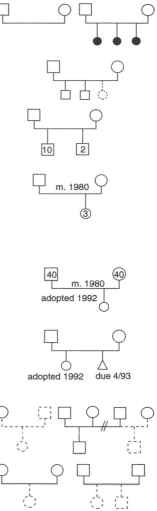

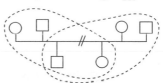

Figure 6.1. Exploring genograms for issues of infertility and involuntary childlessness.

It is apparent when looking at the genograms illustrated in figure 6.1 that there are numerous instances when working with couples, families, single individuals, or gay or lesbian clients that infertility or involuntary childlessness could easily be overlooked without appropriate investigation. Many of the issues illustrated in figure 6.1 can be turned around to become appropriate questions for the alert clinician.

When Children Follow Infertility

Increased Anxiety

When couples decide to postpone childbearing or encounter infertility problems, they may be negatively judged, even by those closest to them. This is still more often the case for women than men, since it is widely accepted that men can show their "credentials" in other ways. When infertile women finally attain the role of parent, they may discover that their parenting activities remain as open to public scrutiny as their struggle with the infertility.

Floyd (1981) reports that when a pregnancy finally occurs, many women feel an increased anxiety level, which sometimes persists into their child's early years. Some even withdraw from sexual relations, fearing that intercourse could somehow endanger the precious fetus; such fears sometimes cause a continued lack of sexual interaction, which precipitates the couple's entering therapy. During therapy, careful exploration of the genogram helps trace the progression of their poor sexual relationship from their infertility through the pregnancy and parenthood stages. The couple is then able to grasp the immense significance of what they have endured and can then finally begin to grapple with an appropriate resolution.

Adaptation to Parenthood

Couples with long histories of infertility, as well as couples who are involuntarily childless, have often expelled parental attitudes, feelings, and abilities from their self-concepts. Once they become parents, through whatever means, it becomes difficult to reintegrate parental roles. As a result, the parent-infant attachment may proceed slowly (Floyd, 1981). Burns (1990) reported that 50 percent of infertile couples indicate varying degrees of bonding difficulty. She also found that these couples report more problems in themselves, their marriages, their parenting, and their children.

The evolution of these family systems is complicated by the fact that the family structure lags behind the developmental needs of the individuals. The partners desired to enter the stage of generativity long before they were able to. They have gone through a redefinition process from a childless state to the tumultuous state of infertility before becoming parents.

Such difficulties may influence the partners to become overattentive parents who manifest difficulty accommodating their child's need for independence (Fulmer, 1989). Glazer and Cooper (1988) state that many of these parents indicate difficulty disciplining their child or children and find it hard to set limits. "This imprint of childlessness not only affects parents' feelings about their children's growth and development but it also has an impact on their behavior" (Glazer & Cooper, p. 216).

Another instance of dysfunctional parenting may occur when the couple becomes disappointed upon discovering that the anticipated rewards are less than the reality. When David and Joan, both in their forties, finally became parents after their third in vitro fertilization, they expected they would always feel the bliss they then experienced. "I used to watch other women in the grocery store," Joan explained one day. "They would be so impatient with their kids. I thought I would never do that. I imagined I would be so happy with this child and appreciate her every moment. I never dreamed I would resent her or feel disappointed or dislike her at times. It makes me feel so guilty."

David became agitated and finally blurted out: "It's more than that Joan. You know you rage at her—you don't just get a little irritated. I cringe when you yell that you hate her. I know she can be defiant sometimes, but she's just a little toddler. She can't help that you're sometimes disappointed in her or disillusioned with your parenting experience."

The research reported by Halman and colleagues (1995), however, contradicts the findings of overanxious parenting. Their research indicated no significant difference between fertile and infertile women regarding their adaption to motherhood. Both infertile and fertile women indicated high levels of coping with the tasks of motherhood. It may be that the infertile women indicate satisfaction with the mothering role and adapt well, but nonetheless remain anxious about it.

The positive adaptation reported by infertile women (Halman, Oakley, & Lederman, 1995) may be related to the high levels of social support for the new mother from family, friends, and significant others, which helps to reduce the stress of postpartum adjustment and assist with carrying out their maternal role. As their marital and family system evolved, these women were able to develop and groom such supports. The secrecy and isolation that many infertile couples resort to during treatment does not seem to inhibit the formation of these significant supports. Perhaps for many of these couples the isolation they experienced during their infertility crisis influences them to actively seek more support during pregnancy and the postpartum period.

Unresolved Couple Conflict

When difficulties arise, the underlying issues may be less related to parenting per se, and more to conflicts left unresolved from the infertile years of the marriage. Marital conflicts can create a family dynamic in which the affections or the conflicts are detoured to the parent-child relationship. The parents may become child-centered in order to avoid conflict with one another. They focus on the parental role at the cost of the spousal role or become overinvested in the child (Burns, 1990). Whereas the infertility was previously triangulated into the marital system, the arrival of the child merely creates a new triangle. The baby's presence then may draw one parent close, leaving the other distant. The child thus becomes an integral part of maintaining family stability. The couple can maintain a semblance of positive feeling regarding the marriage when in fact they are really brushing former disappointments and conflicts away or refocusing through their child-centered existence.

Although parenthood is usually associated with less positive marital exchanges, more conflict, and less leisure time (Halman et al., 1995), parents who have been through infertility report feeling more positive about their marriage after parenthood (Burns, 1990).

A possible explanation may be that the closeness or satisfaction they feel is related to the closeness they feel through the baby rather than an intimacy between them.

When these couples come for therapy focusing on the distance they feel or expressing that the family "just isn't working well together," exploration of the genogram reveals the degree to which their infertility experience has influenced their current difficulties, which often surprises them. With the visual assistance of their genogram, they are presented with a clearer sense of the origins of their difficulties and can more easily focus on ways to put their infertility history in a perspective that is more manageable.

Effects of Family Dynamics on the Child

Such intensity within the family dynamics is overwhelming to the child. The child may exhibit behavior problems such as school failure, truancy, acting out, or physical illness. These children may present for therapy at any developmental stage, even in adulthood, with individuation or differentiation problems. Carey, a 24-year-old accountant, came into therapy because she was having difficulties sustaining relationships. One day she explained, "I always thought my parents were overprotective. I attributed it to the fact that they were older parents and pretty old-fashioned. Then my aunt told me about their infertility. I guess when people have that much trouble having a baby, they must cling to their child more, huh? Anyway, I'm realizing now that I overreact to people—well, to guys—hanging on to me even though they aren't really clinging like my parents did." Carey began to realize that her difficulty with commitment related to her feeling suffocated in her relationship with her parents. She feared that she would similarly feel suffocated or too constrained in a committed relationship with a man. Even though her relationship issues brought her into therapy, it became evident through the exploration of her genogram that her issues were part of the legacy of infertility her parents experienced. When Carey helped create the genogram, she had a context within which to view her parents that included their development as people, marital partners, and parents. Since they had never directly addressed their infertility crisis, they still lived with a sense of crisis in their lives. They reacted to many of Carey's developmental issues in an exaggerated manner rather than realizing she was just trying to test her new wings and was usually not in any real danger. Understanding their context helped Carey find a healthier balance in her own relationships.

Often the parents suffer as much as the children from unresolved conflicts, triangulation, or other dysfunctional family dynamics. A child born to infertile parents is so wanted that the parents often see him or her as "bigger than life" and very special. This creates unreasonably high expectations that he or she will compensate for all the suffering the couple has gone through. In order to continue to create a reliable environment to germinate all of their hopes and aspirations for this child, infertile couples often experience more separation anxiety and thus are often more overprotective, intrusive, and controlling.

Burns (1990) reports that children from families with a legacy of infertility experience more psychosocial and behavioral problems than normally conceived children. It may be that indeed they do experience more problems or it may be that the partners became more used to working together and functioning in concert in order to get through various procedures, and so they continue to parent with the same togetherness. This can lead to overprotectiveness and overscrutiny. Their children may exhibit problems with autonomy or function with more neurotic symptoms. It may also be that as a result of their infertility crisis these parents are more in tune with any developmental difficulties their child faces or are more likely to attribute the problems to the child's origins and to cope with them differently than parents who conceived their children normally. As a result of this increased sensitivity, these parents may be more likely to present for therapy. They focus on the child's behavior, or sometimes on the troubled parent-child relationship, unaware of the continued influence of their infertility experience on their parenting dynamics. When the therapist asks the appropriate questions regarding their decisions about children, spacing of children, or number of children desired, the trauma of infertility is uncovered and further work toward resolution can be achieved.

An alternative way of viewing the overscrutiny may be to reframe the concern these parents exhibit as a positive quality of parenting. The closeness with which the parents interact with the child also provides a warmth and sense of family togetherness. In fact, research conducted by Kovacs, Mushin, Kane, and Baker (1993) indicated no difference in psychosocial development or developmental problems between children conceived through ART and those conceived normally. It is more likely that the parents *perceive* differences that do not actually exist.

WHEN CHILDREN ARE CONCEIVED THROUGH ART

Parenthood achieved through ART, particularly donor egg or sperm insemination, creates another layer of intense emotional impact for couples. When a child is added to a system that endured such a prolonged crisis, the child will of course be affected. The stress may be exacerbated when one of the parents does not share the genetic link with this child. The missing genetic link may pose a threat to the marital relationship or to the relationship between the nongenetic parent and child. An outsider is symbolically infused into the family system, creating asymmetry.

Additionally, if the donor egg or sperm procedure is kept secret, the secret then creates a powerful dynamic within the family system and for the child. There is always something—or someone—that is not spoken about by the parents or within the family. There is a family secret. Developmental issues arise and set off questions or concerns for the parents, who wonder about the genetics but do not speak about any of these questions or concerns. The child may have some sense of the family secret or an unspoken tension between his or her parents, but he or she continues to be deprived of the knowledge. In addition, the child becomes a persistent reminder to the parents of the infertility as well as the narcissistic injury the partners may feel they sustained during this crisis.

The triangle that can be created in the family dynamics through the trauma of the infertility and especially the ART procedures may initially help the child's early growth and development because he or she receives more attention from his or her hovering parents. Eventually such dynamics may create nodal events in the family system that threaten the familiar triangle and thus the homeostasis (Bradt, 1989). The couple, who have been so centered on their infertility, and then their child, now have to look at the fallout from these series of upheavals they have previously ignored.

The Parenting Experience: Tempered with Guilt, Loss, and Grief

GUILT

Infertile women often have difficulty leaving their child in daycare because it reminds them of their childlessness. After the long-anticipated birth, they may choose to remain at home with the child in order to alleviate guilt about leaving the child. Given all they have gone through, how hard they worked to have this child, and how much they wanted this child, they hesitate to relinquish the child's care to a daycare situation. But such intense feelings and their guilt can create more difficult situations. These women experience role conflict as well as role changes. As they struggle with identity issues, they understandably feel some resentment around these changes. They may not feel as competent, in control, or in charge as they did in their offices. Some women may feel they had more respect and were more goal-oriented when they could focus exclusively on their career goals. Or, in retrospect, they may have discovered that the rewards they reaped in their career were more meaningful than they felt at the time, and they now miss such affirmation and challenge. Nodal events create strong emotional reactions as they not only struggle with the rewards of their experiences, of raising this child, but also feel guilty about their resentments.

Similarly, many couples engage in a bargaining process while they are infertile. They will promise never to complain or to resent their child. When these normal feelings arise in the course of parenting or through the new mother's identity struggle, the partners sometimes feel they have made a deal with the devil. Because these spouses worked so hard to get their children, they may feel it is necessary to be a "superparent"; since this is impossible, they feel guilty if the children complain (Eck Menning, 1988). When they feel guilt about not being the perfect parent, they often blame themselves. "When I remember my infertility experience I sometimes feel ashamed, believing it was a sign from God that I would be an unfit mother" (Allen, quoted in Glazer & Cooper, 1988, p. 223). As a result of their guilt and the pressure they place on themselves, these women sometimes feel trapped and may experience an increased incidence of depression, hostility, and interpersonal sensitivity (Burns, 1990).

LOSS

The parents frequently experience an overconcern with loss both because of what they have weathered and because the threat of loss remains real—they fear that something terrible will happen to their child. "Due to the nature of the infertility journey, including the disappointments and disillusionments that appear every step along the way, these losses are not easily repaired, even when a biological child appears at the end of the road" (Cooper & Glazer, 1994, p. 21). In addition, the fact that infertile parents are often older complicates their sense of loss; they are facing other losses simultaneously, such as the loss of their parents, the loss of their own youth through menopause, decreasing physical capabilities or stamina, or even career disappointments.

Just as the ordeal of infertility limits the partners' latitude in expressing frustration or disappointment, so too, as previously mentioned, do they experience mixed feelings surrounding their children's developmental milestones. Although most parents delight in these milestones, they are more threatening for infertile parents because they move the child toward separation. And since infertile parents do not live with the assumption that they can have more children, they are more vulnerable to feelings of loss as they watch their child grow. "We had to leave a restaurant last weekend," explained Alan, a 42-year-old insurance agent. "It was too painful for both of us. We were watching two families with babies next to our table. All we could think about was how quickly Sam had grown up, how much we wanted another baby in our family, and how much we wanted to hold babies again. Sometimes it just seems too hard to have to go through all of this infertility stuff again."

The loss that infertile couples feel can be mediated but not resolved through achieving parenthood. Sometimes they can only acknowledge their loss, disappointment, and the intensity of their struggle after they have attained parenthood or adjusted to nonparenthood.

GRIEF

As with any grief reaction, sometimes the sense of loss is manifested through anger, despair, depression, or denial. However, the grief responses can also affect parenting by inhibiting the growth of close ties; they can also lead to more complicated pathological reactions, which may manifest as denial or conflict and rigidity within the family system. When grief is experienced at such intense levels, it may inhibit appropriate attachment or place pressure on the child to fulfill the template of the wished-for "fantasy" child. When he or she understandably fails to live up to this ideal, abusive or neglectful parenting may result. The family may enter therapy at this point to deal with what they perceive as inadequate parenting due to their failings as parents. Until they work through the historical sequences found in their marital and family genograms, they do not comprehend the significance of their infertility history within the larger scheme of what they are struggling with today.

When Children are Adopted

When a couple has resolved their childlessness through adoption, failure to deal with their unresolved feelings may interfere with their ability to become close to an adopted child or cause them to become overly involved in the child's medical complaints. They may also have difficulty explaining adoption to the child (Sadler & Syrop, 1987).

Although resolution of infertility is a lifelong process, there are two aspects that seem essential. First, the couple needs to give up on the possibility of biological parenthood. The spouses need to mourn their fantasies of their biological child: the beautiful eyes, the musical talent, or the athletic prowess. Second, they need to develop an increased awareness and acceptance of the possibilities of social parenthood through adoption (Matthews & Matthews, 1986). Even though they can ultimately attain the joys of parenthood, they can never erase the struggles, the helplessness, or the pain of their infertility. "Adoptive parents are often startled to find that while their child fulfills much of their need to be a parent, they still feel biologically defective and left out" (Glazer & Cooper, 1988, p. 217).

Contributing to their sense of being different or left out may be a lack of understanding of the adoption process and the adoptive family system within our culture. Adoption carries with it a different set of rituals and meanings (Whiting, 1988). There are few, if any, rituals that have been created to normalize the processes involved in adoption or other alternative methods of creating families. For example, when a couple announces their pregnancy, there is a flurry of activity: the future grandparents quickly come forward to offer a crib or other baby furniture, toys, or other goods and services. Friends do the same and start talking about baby showers. The expectant couple investigates classes that will teach them about birth and early childcare. All of these activities are familiar rituals related to the usual, "normal" processes for creating families. Adoptive families, on the other hand, are left on their own to define this experience and create their own rituals. Although couples frequently tell family and friends that they are attempting to adopt, they do not know when they will actually *have* the baby. They are told by adoption agency personnel not to decorate a baby's room or to prepare in other ways in case their wait will be a long one or the prospective birthparents change their mind at the last minute. So, they do not have rituals in terms of preparing for the baby. They also do not experience the rituals of pregnancy: feeling the baby kick or seeing her during an ultrasound. Nor do they have clearly established rituals to welcome the baby when they finally do take possession of her. Given that these families already feel great loss and perhaps defective or left out of the mainstream, the need for rituals seems significant. However the challenge to create these rituals becomes one more hurdle these already stressed systems have to surmount. Instead of being able to depend on familiar rituals to bring comfort, they have to push themselves to be creative, to construct something meaningful out of the sterile void of infertility. The adoptive family's ability to create their own meanings, however, would contribute to resolution and the healing of the family system.

Lifelong Childlessness

Some couples resolve their infertility with a decision to become child-free. Sara and Eric, both high-powered corporate attorneys, never dreamed they would have problems reaching any of their goals, especially their goal of starting a family. Their involuntary childlessness forced them to undergo a transition from the anticipated status of potential parenthood to the unwanted status of nonparenthood. They needed to adapt and reorganize on a number of new levels.

"Our terrible experiences with the infertility forced us to reexamine our motives, our need for a child," explained Eric one session. "We just said this was taking too high of a toll on our lives. We realized how much we loved our cats and how easy it was to find a cat sitter and continue to travel, go out to dinner, and buy ourselves new toys. We realized more and more the level of trade-offs and decided maybe it wouldn't be awful to consider not having our own child. In fact, we realized that we just had different kinds of children."

Eric was referring to the notion of alternative methods of experiencing generativity other than parenting. Some couples invent meaningful ways of creating through hobbies or projects. Eric and Sara built their own ski chalet, "a true dream-house" as Eric labeled it. Some individuals express their generativity through creative endeavors like painting, or mastering a new activity, such as gourmet cooking, tennis or horseback riding. Although it is a viable and certainly a necessary option, "voluntary childlessness is a particularly distinctive behavior in a society such as ours which is traditionally pronatalist" (Gutman, 1985). Although infertile couples do not initially choose a child-free existence, they often experience criticism from those who are not familiar with their history and pain. Their decision, of course, evolved through a long and arduous process. For them it is a healthy culmination of that process and all of the accompanying misery.

Couples should have the freedom to choose their family configuration based on what works for them, rather than on pressures from the larger culture. Gutman (1985) discusses the descriptions of the typology of couples who have decided to be childless. As she explains, it is ironic that descriptors such as hedonistic, idealistic, or practical are frequently used to categorize couples who are childless. Such negative biases often confront even those couples choosing a child-free existence following infertility. Upon explanation, many find understanding or support. The larger problem, however, is that most people judge and feel free to comment without any knowledge of the painful sequence of events and the laborious subsequent decision-making process.

The rapid growth of medical technology and treatment possibilities "has increased the belief that a baby at any price is acceptable" (Burns, 1990, p. 187). Therefore, most couples, like Sara and Eric, not only begin their journey with the goal of child bearing and rearing, but also continue to hold out hope and persevere. Seeking medical treatment "serves to objectify what had previously been only a personal and subjective reality" (Matthews & Matthews, 1986, p. 643). Couples who remain infertile and childless without a clear diagnosis encounter the strongest social and psychological consequences. It is as if they remain in a limbo state, still hopeful yet puzzled, feeling cheated and empty, yet not confronting a clear ending point in their road. Their infertility represents an involuntary and not easily reversible state. The prospect of lifelong childlessness remains too difficult for these individuals to consider.

Coping with lifelong childlessness is further complicated by the fact that infertility represents a number of losses at many different levels. The grief work has to encompass issues around the loss of a desired child, a genetic heir, loss of the assumption of parenthood and the concommitant life plans and goals. The grief itself has long-term effects associated with childlessness or possible losses through miscarriage or the adoption that fell through.

Careful exploration of the genogram can extract these issues even though couples may most likely present with alternative issues. They may also present for therapy with puzzlement over "this sudden sense of sadness in my life" when in fact the depression relates to an "anniversary" reaction. In other words, the mere passage of time cannot account for a couple's adjustment, or lack of adjustment, to their infertility experience. A seemingly sudden reawakening of anger or grief could occur a year or more later. It could be a significant date the couple had not consciously noted, such as the date of their IVF transfer or the date of the menstrual period when they discovered the high-tech solution did not result in the desired pregnancy.

For some couples, the anniversary reaction becomes the turning point at which they are finally able to move on. The resolution for some will of course be alternative methods of becoming parents, such as adoption or surrogacy. Others may decide to continue their lives without adding a child to their couple system. They may find other ways to be involved with children, through Big Brother or Big Sister programs, for example, or with nieces and nephews. Or like Sara and Eric, they may become child-free though a conscious and deliberate sorting process.

Implications for Therapy

When infertility is not the presenting complaint, it can be difficult for the therapist, and certainly for the couple, to identify the actual source of their pain, their unhappiness, or sense of lack of control. As they explore their marital and family of origin histories through the use of the genogram, it can become evident that much of their sorrow or anger relates to their unresolved infertility. They may still be childless rather than child-free or they may need to resume their discussions about alternative methods of achieving parenthood. Asking the relevant questions about their histories will illuminate these unresolved issues:

- Ask about any health-related issues, including miscarriages.
- Have they thought about or do they plan to have children?
- Were their children anticipated or planned at specific times?
- If the client is single, has he or she ever been in—or is he or she now in—a long-term committed relationship?
- If single, how do they feel about having, or not having children in their life?

Understandably, most couples have trouble deciding to end treatment. Some just continue to periodically talk about further interventions, but do not actively set up appointments. Others explore alternatives, such as adoption, without ever articulating whether they believe they are finished with the medical treatments. In their research, Freeman and colleagues (1987) noted that only about half of the women they interviewed definitively indicated they had terminated treatment; about 20 percent remained undecided about continuing treatments.

The emotional upheaval created for couples who experience long-term struggles with infertility or for those couples living in limbo is enormous. These couples have to redefine their reality at various points along the path. Because infertility changes their view of reality, it significantly influences their self-concept and identity. Since the infertile couple sought to define their future identities as parents, the infertility crisis precipitates identity shock (Matthews & Matthews, 1986). The shock is more difficult for couples who perceive a biological solution as the only solution. A woman "may have formed her whole identity around the idea that she would one day marry and bear children. When this is denied her, she may feel totally unemployed even though she may work at a career she enjoys. She sees her identity as a woman as incomplete" (Eck Menning, 1988, p. 105).

"I didn't fully realize until I actually saw this picture, this genogram thing, that all of my terrible feelings are related to our infertility, to my sense of emptiness," explained Marcy, a 38-year-old medical technician. "I feel like I live in this bubble, like I'm always on the outside looking in at all these normal people who are just going about their lives. They have their children, they go to the grocery, and they have a family to celebrate Christmas with. I just don't know where I belong anymore."

Her husband, Alex, a 37-year-old physical therapist, reacted strongly. "It isn't just an issue for Marcy. I feel lots of upheaval too. I wanted to have kids, to be a family. I'm angry about living in this limbo. I thought we would be somewhere else in our lives by now."

Since child bearing and rearing are closely tied to role fulfillment and identity, the crisis may have a greater effect on a man or woman's social identity than many other types of stigma. The partners need to redefine the situation so that their goals become more congruent with the possible alternatives. Once Marcy and Alex understood the source of their problems, they could look more vigorously at the medical and nonmedical options. She and her husband were ready to hear more action-oriented solutions which channeled their strong emotions into productive avenues. They were ultimately able to stand firm in their conviction that they were no longer willing to live in limbo, that they wanted to work toward becoming child-free and moving on with life.

Since infertility is not simply resolved with the advent of a pregnancy, some couples tend to be overly anxious about the pregnancy itself, childbirth, and subsequent parenthood. Such anxiety at any of these junctures may be the presenting issue for therapy and a clue that it may be related to a history of infertility. It is useful to support the couple throughout the pregnancy as well as postpartum to help with the transition to parenthood. Understandings the couple gleans in therapy can mitigate a tendency toward overprotectiveness or reduce the potential of becoming overly child-centered to the detriment of the couple relationship. Urge the partners to find time for communicating and playing together, even sexually, in order to become focused on each other again. Therapy can provide further grief work for one or both partners to move beyond previous miscarriage experiences, for example, or a needed forum in which to explore the many intense feelings they have been struggling with throughout their infertility and the treatments. Couples often need to talk about their sense of lack of control, which may be exacerbated by a newborn. Discussing specific ways of gaining some control over their new lives can be helpful.

- Asking how they manifest control in other areas of their lives helps them realize strengths they already have and then to look at how they might generalize these to this aspect of their lives.
- Helping them look for ways to nurture each other and themselves is important as they are struggling with other new challenges, the stresses of parenting, lack of sleep, and the changing relationships with friends and families of origin as they formulate their own nuclear family.
- Helping them structure some specific routines, even if they are new ones, gives them a sense of increased control.

Couples who have not achieved a viable pregnancy need to look at their current goals. Spouses may present for therapy with specific issues or just a sense of meaninglessness in their lives or in their marriage. During the genogram exploration, issues stemming from their infertility and their unclear goals surrounding parenting will become more apparent to them. At this point, the therapist can focus her questions to help them assess their desires for parenting and begin to refine their goals. If they seem set on becoming parents, will that entail further medical intervention or other measures? Do they really want to commit to such challenges? If they still feel strong wishes for the parenting experience, but do not want further medical challenges, they need to begin discussing when to quit the medical options and concentrate their energies elsewhere. Perhaps they are ready to accept the possibility of social rather then biological parenthood though adoption. This requires a redefinition of self and self as parent, but can lead to a healthy resolution of their infertility. If adoption becomes their goal, the therapist can direct them to specific adoption resources, such as adoption agencies or lawyers who specialize in adoption services.

Regardless of the path couples take to achieve parenthood, they often attempt to compensate for all of their difficulties by becoming superparents. This simply prolongs the pain of infertility by emphasizing how they are different rather than how they are similar to other families. They will have the same feelings of resentment and frustration as those who more easily became parents. These couples must be encouraged, even pushed, to identify and label their feelings of anger, times of frustration, or their disappointments about their parenting experience. Since it is usual to then feel guilt about these feelings, they must be urged to articulate that. They need permission to have such feelings, despite the hurdles they had to navigate to attain parenthood. Since parenthood is not as blissful as they had fantasized, normalizing their feelings can be of great help in their continued adjustment to parenthood and the resolution of the infertility.

Sometimes exploration of the genogram and the right questions can illuminate the causes of a couple's inability to mobilize following IVF or other treatment failures or a miscarriage. Often the couple or a partner simply describes depression or malaise when presenting for therapy. One or both may realize an increased sensitivity to grief or feelings of sadness in their life without making the connection with the infertility or treatment failures. Helping them label how much they have been through and reassuring them that they have done all that is medically possible for them at this time bring some healing. Grief and mourning are necessary and healthy aspects of resolving their infertility; therefore it is important to explore whether the grief is related to premature termination of treatment, treatment that was not successful, or whether they find it difficult to grieve fully and openly because they are uncertain about seeking more medical intervention. Helping the couple examine how and what they might learn from this difficult experience aids their grieving process. The therapist's acknowledgment that the issues infertile couples have experienced don't diminish once they become parents is a strong message to these struggling couples that they are not aberrant. They have indeed survived a crisis and unless the issues related to the crisis are addressed, they will have difficulty moving beyond it. They become more capable of focusing on how and where to put energy in other areas of their lives. These couples have many strengths and resources—after all, they are the characteristics that allowed them to survive the many infertility hurdles and that subsequently helped them brave the challenges of therapy. Even if they did not consciously realize what brought them to this point and to the therapy, their marital system was strong enough to weather the crises and move ahead.

7

INVOLUNTARILY CHILDLESS BUT NOT NECESSARILY INFERTILE

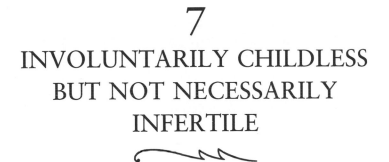

UNIMAGINED ADVANCES in medical technology, coupled with major cultural and political changes for women, have precipitated the growth and increased visibility and viability of variant family forms. The increase in divorce and subsequent blended family configurations have changed the definition of the traditional family. Simultaneously, many women have postponed marriage due to increased career options and an emphasis on self-development and career development. As they have become more respected in the employment arena and are able to advance professionally, they find it more difficult to meet single men who are their intellectual equals or who are simply "right" for them (Pakizegi, 1990).

Regardless of the extent of such demographic and cultural change, children and parenting are still desired by most women. The categorization of family life stages into periods of family of origin and family of procreation attests to the ingrained cultural expectations about parenthood. With such strong messages, it is easy to understand the pain experienced by singles and those in alternative family forms who are excluded from parenthood. In fact, the cultural imperative is so powerful that "involuntary childlessness and nonparenthood are likely to have as significant an impact on family and personal identities as parenthood itself" (Matthews & Matthews, 1986, p. 645). The missing link to the next generation often becomes a driving force for childless singles or couples, who frequently pursue all avenues of medical and social options in order to fulfill this desire.

The strong cultural mandate regarding marriage, parenting, and family seems to be more harshly directed toward women then men. Childless women are criticized more than childless men (Stewart & Robinson, 1989). The cultural stereotypes of single women include accusations that they are not capable of forming relationships with men or that no men are interested in them, they are lesbians or feminists, emotionally disturbed, or just plain selfish. The reality is that most single women are heterosexual and hope to marry in the future (Pakizegi, 1990).

It is ironic that many childless individuals are negatively regarded because they do not conform to society's view of the traditional family. Those outside of the individual's world have no idea that the childlessness may be involuntary. Singles who desire children experience a great deal of pain with the emptiness in their home and their hearts. They would like a partner, but the lack of a child is frequently even more painful. Some women have divorced husbands who didn't want children and now find themselves without a partner and without a child. Yet the biological clock keeps ticking. So, some of these women—and their male counterparts—begin to consider single parenthood.

Advances in reproductive technology and societal changes have given single women choices regarding their careers, their bodies, and their lifestyles. This includes the opportunity to create variations in the family or parenting themes. A major hurdle, however, is self-doubt, fueled by the questions and judgments of society. Because they are viewed as different, selfish, or peculiar, they are also frequently labeled as not fit for parenthood. Additionally, "When single women or lesbian couples opt for ovum donation, especially if they are older, they are creating families that are even more nontraditional" (Cooper & Glazer, 1994, p. 208). Cultural prejudices about single women are often shared by medical personnel, who may feel uncomfortable with this population. Not surprisingly, single fatherhood is also seen by some as an aberration and single fathers often have a harder time psychologically and socially (Tauer, 1996).

The suspicions and biases of society and the larger culture have not been substantiated, however. Arguments have been made in the literature that there are no a priori reasons to exclude single and lesbian couples from the assisted reproduction programs. Studies of nontraditional families have identified some variables that predict good adjustment and some unique strengths that children from these families manifest (Barwin, 1993; Cramer, 1986; Gibbs, 1988; Jacob, in press). Additionally, since their lifestyle includes interactions in community schools and with friends who live in two-parent heterosexual families, they experience interactions with the larger, more traditional culture. Obviously, these variables have been important ones, since children from these variant families are faring well (Jacob, in press).

Statistically, the number of nontraditional families has increased. For example, the number of children living with never-married mothers during the period from 1980 through 1985 increased from 1.8 million to 3.5 million, an increase of almost 100 percent (Statistical Abstracts, 1987). Also, 1970 to 1984 marked the greatest increase in births to single women over 30 (Pakizegi, 1990). The 1980s also witnessed a lesbian baby boom, with an estimated 6 to 14 million children growing up in approximately 4 million gay and lesbian households (Keedle, 1994). It can be seen that more people are taking advantage of major societal shifts to create these unique family forms.

Most people find it difficult to clearly articulate why they want a child. The reasons are complex and emotional. Technically, the right to bear or have children should be as available to those who wish parenthood as any other right in our society. Single and gay or lesbian individuals, however, are often required to articulate their desires more extensively than the married heterosexual population. Since one- to two-thirds of single women seeking parenthood through assisted reproduction were previously married, it seems questionable to object merely on the basis of present marital status. The person has not changed; she is still the same woman with the same family of origin issues and the same personality dynamics. In some cases she may have even divorced in order to have a child if her husband could not or would not have a child.

An individual contemplating such procedures experiences tremendous turmoil in view of the fact that the medical procedures and the "family" are nontraditional. The decision to proceed is generally a well-considered one. The process involves first assessing the security of employment, then insuring adequate social support, and finally assessing emotional readiness. Since the biological clock is quickly ticking, the above considerations are only part of the equation. A further set of decisions may need to be made regarding the use of biologically assisted reproduction, donor insemination, or the adoption options.

Singles

"I just assumed I'd get married and have my kids like my Mom and my sister did," explained Linda, a 32-year-old teacher. "Now I am being interrogated like a criminal just because I want that kid and don't have the husband to go with it." Linda was referring to the lengthy evaluation process she was encountering prior to her requested donor insemination procedure. "It isn't that I don't want a husband—I would love to be married like my best friends, but that just hasn't happened. The problem is, I know how desperately I want a kid and I just can't wait much longer."

Although many women desire to marry in the future, they experience a sense of urgency and begin to realize they desire motherhood more than marriage. Although many women no longer apologize for not having a husband, they often still feel a need to provide excuses for their "failure" to have children. They, as well as their family, consider childlessness as inappropriate. Ironically, they very much desire children in their lives. Those who are involuntarily childless, "unlike the voluntarily childless, . . . have generally assumed that becoming parents was part of the process of adult family life" (Matthews & Matthews, 1986, p. 641). They feel tricked, betrayed, and almost ashamed by their childlessness.

For many singles, especially women, their thirtieth birthday becomes a motivating force in their decision to seek parenthood. Even if they are in a relationship, those who decide to request donor insemination do not consider this or any past relationship sufficiently stable or loving to warrant shared parenting (McCartney, 1985). They also feel more rootedness and stability in their lives at this life stage and so as a result feel more comfortable exploring their reproductive options. As expected, numerous women also choose to explore their adoption options. For many this is a more comfortable option, since it is a more familiar societal phenomenon. Women choosing adoption are also influenced by the realization that they are approaching the end of their fertile years. Most are highly educated and financially comfortable and able to choose their options, but desire a nonbiological alternative (Pakizegi, 1990).

Although single men do not experience the same sense of urgency surrounding the biological clock issues, they also often desire to become parents. For men in our culture, however, generativity is not restricted to biological fatherhood. In fact, Snarey (1988) found that infertile men who had adopted had the highest rates of creative, generative activities, even more extensive than infertile men who became biological fathers or fertile men. These men found new ways of adding meaning to their life, such as learning a new hobby, building a summer home, taking classes in a subject that interested them, starting their own business, or developing an extensive project at work. So, although many men have the same desires as women to experience parenthood as a means to transit through this developmental stage, "parenthood of any form appears to be foundation though not an absolute guarantee of reaching this life cycle stage" (Snarey, p. 62). Traditionally, it has been more acceptable for men to experience generativity through other avenues, particularly their careers.

Regardless of how these single men and women ultimately decide to deal with this developmental stage, the decision about how or what to do is most often an arduous one, lasting an average of four years (Mechaneck, Klein, & Kuppersmith, 1988). Historically, it was assumed that single women conceived by accident or carelessness. However, research indicates that more often it has been a carefully considered decision. According to Jacob (in press), for women going through donor insemination procedures, age and emotional readiness are key factors in deciding when to proceed.

As the profile of single mothers by choice continues to emerge, the composition of this group seems to be educated women with an average age of 39 (Jacob, in press). They value being actively involved in shaping their own lives and are persistent in pursuing goals related to their relationships and careers. They perceive themselves as independent and competent, thus quite able to manage the roles of provider and parent. These women "represent a new and separate phenomenon from the classic unwed mother who was generally poor, a teenager, unprepared for motherhood and socially ostracized" (Mechaneck et al., 1988, p. 263).

Mechaneck and colleagues (1988) examined some differences between singles choosing motherhood and those choosing a more traditional path of marriage, formation of the couple relationship, and then motherhood. They found that women choosing more traditional paths had better relationships with their own mothers throughout childhood and adolescence. Compared to married women, singles choosing motherhood described their fathers more negatively. It makes sense that these singles may be willing to forego a relationship with a man, even though they are not willing to forego parenthood.

Available Options

For women choosing biological parenthood, the method of conception employed is often not the original one desired (Mechaneck et al., 1988). They encounter obstacles such as the inability to find a willing partner, resistance by the medical community to perform donor insemination procedures for singles, or difficulty conceiving.

Donor insemination is a popular choice for women who desire to experience pregnancy or for those who desire a sense of control over their bodies. These women are also comfortable with the reality of parenting without a partner. They know they do not have to worry about an accidental conception and they do not entertain any fantasies that the biological father would develop an active interest in the child.

Part of the decision to seek insemination procedures is whether to seek a known or unknown donor. Some women choose to actively pursue pregnancy with a known donor, with or without his knowledge. Those who work out a reproductive relationship with an informed, consenting male confront problems if they have difficulty conceiving immediately. If they suspect infertility, they are even more hesitant to ask their male friend because of the anticipated need for prolonged cooperation (McCartney, 1985). If they are infertile or do not conceive right away, they have to prolong his involvement and worry about possible complications with the continued involvement.

Many women discard the idea of pregnancy with a nonconsenting male for moral reasons. Lesbian women often find the option of pursuing pregnancy with a known donor—with or without his consent—distasteful, and may feel it violates fidelity vows. Women who do seek a known donor must decide whether to work inside the medical system. Such a decision may be dictated by concerns regarding infertility. If attempting to conceive with a known donor, these concerns demand open and frank communication about the man's expectations. If medical personnel are involved, they can help the woman and man execute a written plan that includes each partner's intentions should a pregnancy occur. Sadly, those who have visions of the biological father's involvement may be disappointed and embittered because few remain in the picture after the baby is born (Mechaneck et al., 1988). To some extent, the contract may mitigate some of the disappointment or anger.

Although many single women desire to experience a pregnancy, many also consider adoption. Adoption is still the most widely accepted avenue for singles to achieve parenthood, probably because it has a long history and is viewed by many as an act of altruism (Mechaneck et al., 1988). Many adoption agencies readily accept singles but not lesbian or gay couples, or they offer only children with special needs since these placements traditionally have been viewed as less desirable. Paradoxically, however, such placements require even more emotional and financial assets, which further exhaust the individual's or couple's resources.

Taking into account the complicated medical and relationship issues, adoption becomes a less complicated option for single men to attain parenthood. Ironically, these men frequently receive conflicting messages. On the one hand, friends reinforce how wonderful they are because they took on such a big responsibility; on the other, they are just as frequently given unsolicited advice about fatherhood. "Adoptive fathers in particular may be treated as incompetent caregivers, while at the same time being extolled as models for other men" (Melina, 1986, p. 224).

A big problem for these men and women, however, is that they encounter intense competition for adopted children and are often told their unmarried status will be a disadvantage. Although singles are accepted by many countries for international adoptions, they are not as readily accepted for domestic adoptions. In identified adoptions, where the birthparents choose a particular home situation from agency records, they seek a family situation—two parents—since they cannot provide this for their child. In spite of all of these hurdles, single adoptive parents are experiencing as much success as married couples in the raising of their children (Melina, 1986).

Regardless of how single mothers by choice achieve parenthood, most are happy with their decision and positive about their experience of motherhood. They do admit, however, that it is important for the single mother to be realistic about the ways a child can challenge her lifestyle. Mothers find it difficult to set aside time for dating—and find that many men are not interested in the child. This is compounded by the additional cost of childcare for social time and guilt about being away from the child. "I met this great guy at a party," explained Marie, a 34-year-old nail technician who had built a thriving nail salon over the past five years. "We talked most of the night. He was so easy to talk to. Then, when he asked me out he seemed turned off to find out I had to get a babysitter for my little girl. You know, it's so lonely sometimes. I like my life, my career, and my motherhood, and I love my little princess, but I just feel isolated sometimes and would like a companion—a guy—in my life too."

Financial stress is one of the most significant negative stressors reported by single mothers. In fact, most indicate that they want more than one child but that it is not possible due to financial reasons (Jacob, 1997; Pakizegi, 1990). Costs of housing, transportation, and childcare in single-parent families are estimated to be 5 percent higher than for two-parent households (Tauer, 1996). This may be partially due to the fact that single mothers require childcare not only during work hours, but also in order to run errands, attend to business commitments or business travel, and perhaps for some social time.

Other negative aspects single parents experience include feeling tremendous stress from performing multiple roles with no adult backup, feeling chronically tired, encountering a lack of understanding from bosses or coworkers who don't grasp the urgency of retrieving a child from childcare on time, and being the only accountable adult in that child's life in the case of an emergency. An employment situation can create a great deal of additional stress because, as a sole provider, job security is crucial. Both single fathers and mothers feel this stress when employers or coworkers look askance at their inflexible exit schedule. "I can't help it," cried Helen during one session. "I have to leave when I have to leave. My boss sometimes just stands there with a glare, but his wife is home with his kids all day. I have to pick up Emily on time or I get charged extra. And I don't want the daycare people angry with me. If they drop me and Emily, I'm doomed." Some of these men and women also pass up opportunities for management jobs or other advancement because they can't risk future downsizing, which could eliminate their job or jeopardize their financial security.

In addition to the pressures from employment situations, some single mothers experience negative societal judgments of themselves and their children. It is useful to remember, however, that the advent of the single parent by choice is still a relatively new phenomenon. Historically, the child of an unmarried woman was considered an outcast with limited legal rights; there were standard societal biases about the absent father that produced questions about a child's potential psychological problems or moral development. Interestingly though, research by Mechaneck and colleagues (1988) indicates that today few single mothers experience social ostracism, although some experience disapproval from parents and co-workers.

Lesbian and Gay Couples

Single men and women creating variant family forms through adoption or donor insemination procedures enjoy both legal and social sanctions. However, even though the law recognizes biological parents, stepparents, and adoptive parents, in most states the law does not currently recognize homosexual partners as legitimate parents. For example, the legitimacy of a child born to a heterosexual couple through donor insemination is protected under state law in Connecticut, but such legitimate protection is not afforded lesbian or gay couples. Similarly, although adoption agencies have discretion, "the prevailing bias ... is to prefer married couples over single people, and heterosexuals over lesbians and gay men" (Connecticut Women's Education and Legal Fund, 1995, p. 49).

Therefore, when gay or lesbian individuals make the decision to become parents, the process often restimulates old feelings regarding their deprivileged status. They have to struggle with the emptiness of childlessness as well as stark reminders of their distinctive differences. Even though most therapists would hope that a family would be defined by love and not blood, the facts that these individuals may be very good parents and greatly desire parenthood are not sufficient to overcome many societal biases. Lesbians and gay men who want to present their relationships openly are managing to adopt, but the options are limited. Laws in New York and California legally protect against discrimination in adoption. Thirteen states specifically allow single lesbians or gay men to adopt, although only one partner can be the parent on record (Kantrowitz, 1996). Florida and New Hampshire prohibit these adoptions and other states do not have laws that specifically protect or preclude homosexual adoptions (Martin, 1993). Many adoption agencies are aware that lesbians or gay men present themselves as singles, at least initially, in order to avoid potential discrimination. In these instances, the lesbian or gay man must struggle with the issue of deception or the potential threat of ultimately jeopardizing the adoption finalization. All of these considerations must be weighed against the possibility of being dismissed in the early stages because of discrimination.

Although most people go through considerable deliberations before committing to parenthood and most experience ambivalence about parenting as well as the extraordinary commitment involved, single and lesbian women find it hard to acknowledge these feelings. They also feel more obligated than marrieds might to justify their choice. Because they struggle with being different, they feel that in many ways they have to be smarter or better and certainly as well adjusted—if not above and beyond—their heterosexual counterparts. Lesbian women traverse through five stages in choosing to become mothers (Loulan, in Jacob, in press, p. 10):

1. Initially, they merely realize that it is a possible option for them.
2. They recognize that it is an attractive option, but one that may not be right for them.
3. In the third stage, they don't yet feel ready even though they know it can now be a possibility in their lives.
4. As they move into the fourth stage, they come to terms with being ready and begin to plan for parenthood.
5. Finally, they create a plan and deliberately decide to act on this carefully constructed plan.

During these stages, these women struggle with many of the same factors single women struggle with, such as issues of financial stability or whether good social support will be available from family and friends. Although they are aware of their need for these supports, they also recognize their own strengths, such as their ability to be goal-oriented and independent.

The next significant step often involves making the decision about who will bear the child. Sometimes only one partner desires to bear the child or experience childbirth, or only one partner may be biologically able to conceive or carry the pregnancy. Sometimes the decision is simply based on the anticipated reactions of each partner's family. "We just knew that Sandy's parents would be horrified if she were pregnant. We knew her parents would go crazy if they had to face their relatives and friends to explain her pregnant, unmarried state," explained Melissa, a 36-year-old physician. "On the other hand, my parents, especially my mom, and even my sister will probably be ecstatic to have a baby in the family. My parents are also okay with the fact that I'm lesbian and they like Sandy." Other lesbian couples must also struggle with age-related considerations or health insurance coverage issues, which present additional and sometimes stressful considerations.

The decision about who will biologically carry the child is only one of many for these couples. They also have to struggle with decisions regarding how to achieve the pregnancy. If they have decided to attempt biological parenthood rather than adoption, they then turn to donor insemination procedures. Kate, a 38-year-old optometrist, worked out a complex agreement with her gay friend James. "James told me he always wanted children," she told me one session, "so one day I just asked him if he wanted to father a child. I liked him a lot and thought it would be fine to have him involved. So we worked out the visitation and financial agreements. It's been great to have another parent there."

Even though Kate was fond of James and their relationship didn't involve the complications a partner would entail, she still requested insemination procedures because it was disagreeable to both her and James to have intercourse. She also felt safer in terms of protecting both of them from the potential of disease. According to Jacob (1997), 5000 to 10,000 children are born to lesbian couples through donor insemination or planned intercourse. Although Kate's situation worked well for her and James, many lesbian singles and couples favor an anonymous donor so as not to have the complicated involvement with the biological father.

Regardless of the complexity of the decisions about who will bear the child or the method of impregnation, the pregnancy itself sets off power imbalances in the relationship. Although this is true in heterosexual relationships to some degree, it is more problematic in lesbian relationships because of the relationship dynamics. First, there exists the potential possibility that either partner could carry the pregnancy. Second, since a high degree of closeness, rather than differentiation, is usually more characteristic of lesbian relationships, the introduction of another player, a child, threatens the fused connection the partners have thus far enjoyed. Additionally, if the biological father is known, his presence, whether actual or symbolic, creates a triangle, again threatening the intimacy and connectedness of the couple system.

To complicate the picture even further, lesbian couples have to cope with the cultural definition that a child has only one mother. Lesbian couples sometimes seek to rectify this situation by creating the concept of a "co-mother," which functionally works as a two-parent family system. Any difficulty is most likely to occur when deciding who will provide which parenting functions and deciding how the child will address each of the parents. With no traditional gender roles to fall back on, everyone pitches in with household tasks, but this does not resolve the issue surrounding how to address the parent figures. Also, since the biological mother may have functioned in her intimate relationships in a closely connected manner, she may also, consciously or not, fuse with the child and find it difficult to share this intimacy, some of the parenting, or even the power. Meanwhile, the co-mother struggles with her sense of being an invisible parent within this family, or with the school, the pediatrician, and perhaps even within her own family of origin.

Gay men struggle with somewhat different issues as they consider parenthood. Lyle, a 37-year-old architect, and Charlie, a 38-year-old family therapist, decided they wanted to parent two children. They had been partners for eight years and felt they really wanted to be a family. After much deliberation, and researching the various options and state statutes, they chose to adopt two females—an infant and a toddler—from South America. "We agreed that we really wanted two children," explained Lyle, "and we argued about whether or not to attempt a biological route, but we really felt it would be too complicated and might entail too much legal hassle or risk."

For gay men who wish to be the primary parents to a child biologically related to them, surrogacy is the only route open to them. Although some gay men or couples are lucky enough to have very good female friends who might consider carrying their child, such a case is not usual. Surrogacy can present difficult legal entanglements. "Courts are reluctant to terminate parental rights of women who bear children for men, even in cases where the women have agreed to relinquish their parental rights" (Connecticut Women's Education and Legal Fund, 1995). Even in California, a state often considered somewhat friendly to gays and lesbians, the courts uphold surrogacy as not enforceable. The New Jersey courts condemn surrogacy as the sale of a child. Although Michigan opened the door to limited surrogacy possibilities, the arrangement would not include the surrogate's surrender of parental rights. So even though Lyle and Charlie were eventually able to adopt their two little girls, it involved considerable research, some compromise, particularly regarding a biologically related child, and more difficulty than their heterosexual friends encountered with the same agency.

Although lesbian and gay couples affirm their nontraditional family status in a sexist and homophobic world, the children growing up in these families have more similarities than differences when compared to children from heterosexual families. In fact, the usual concern that these children would be ostracized and teased has not been the case. Studies researching these issues have not supported the hypothesis that these children would experience more life problems (Jacob, 1995).

The parenthood experience is a very positive one for these individuals. They feel more connected to their community and are often more active as a result. For some, having a child also helps repair strained family relationships, since most grandparents find it difficult to remain distant from their grandchildren even if they can distance from their gay or lesbian children.

Out-of-Phase Couples

Singles, lesbians, and gays are not alone in the struggle to swim against the tide, to be atypical, and to wish for children and a "normal" family life. Many heterosexual couples who would be considered within the realm of traditional and "normal" because of their couple status, in fact experience a sense of being aberrant when it comes to issues regarding children. "When Rick and I first got together," Melanie, a 41-year-old lawyer, explained one session, "I was very careful about not getting pregnant. In fact, my best friend, Kelly, got pregnant and had an abortion. It was just so important to all of us to get ahead and put all our energies into our careers. Now Rick has no interest or energy for this whole kid thing. Somehow many of my friends have kids in high school already, so again I'm out of sync."

The elongated professional model (Fulmer, 1989), which Melanie has described, creates a variant structure within the larger culture. Many young, well-educated professionals postpone childbearing so long that some can then have only a small number of children or are confronted with infertility problems. Sadly, once these successful high-powered people decide to have children, they face disappointment and a feeling of helplessness they have not previously encountered.

Somehow these couples were just humming along like well-tuned instruments until one partner woke up one day and wished to alter their marital course. They had looked to their careers and their marriage as a "distinctive private world over which they have some control and which they can shape to some extent" (Matthews & Matthews, 1986, p. 643). Now, of course, they feel betrayed by life and their expectations, and angry about the course they had pursued. "I sure enjoy being with Rick and talking to him about things, but a big part of why I got married was to eventually have a family," Melanie lamented one day. "I just wonder now, if we don't have kids, what will give us meaning? I guess I'm asking what will give *me* meaning?"

Melanie had understandably assumed that her marriage would provide her with companionship, children, and security. Instead, because of their delayed childbearing and potential childlessness, she and her husband have a situation of which they can make no sense. She and Rick were harshly confronted with a major reconstruction of reality—of the life reality they assumed they would ultimately achieve. The prolonged first phase of their marriage and the postponement of having children pushed them into an out-of-phase mode.

Special Issues for Remarried Partners

Remarried couples often feel out of sync with one another as well as with the more traditional culture. The research indicates that almost 20 percent of the couples requesting in vitro fertilization have biological or stepchildren and a smaller percent already have an adopted child (Mazure & Greenfield, 1989). Indeed, a couple's endeavors to form their own ideal family often creates the impetus for discussion about another child. "When we married I wasn't sure I wanted a child," explained Joy, a 42-year-old librarian. "We were quite involved with Alan's kids and we were all very close then. All of our friends had kids about the same ages so we had quite a social network too. I was so delighted to finally have a big, happy family, like in the movies. How could I have anticipated their mother moving across the country with them so that we could hardly be involved with them? All of a sudden I just felt so empty."

As Joy began to lobby for another child, Alan began to withdraw from her. They did not totally comprehend the degree of loss Alan was feeling. While he was still acutely mourning the loss of his own children, he found it extremely difficult to increase the intensity of his relationship with Joy. Similarly, it was too painful for Alan to entertain being vulnerable to yet another child. He was also clear that he had satisfied his need for generativity in an earlier life stage. "I miss my kids terribly much," he said tearfully one session, "but that doesn't make me want to have another one now. I've been there. I know how much this means to Joy, but we have to be realistic about our age, our careers, earning power, and, you know, where we are in our lives."

Alan had been influenced by his best friend and tennis partner, David, who had remarried and created another family. "I'm too old for this baby-up-at-night stuff," David told him one week. "And then I'm up another night with my son who just started driving. Boy, I never knew two different kids and two different situations could present such exhausting challenges." However, David's situation, regardless of difficulty, is somewhat common.

David and his second wife, Allison's, situation was somewhat different from Alan and Joy's. David had a 7-year-old son when he began to date Allison, who was a young, never-married associate in his firm. Allison had been clear when they were dating that she wanted to have her own children, even though she had a good relationship with David's son. Both David and Alan agreed that the honeymoon was over too soon with their new spouses. "It's so hard to stay positive about each other when you have fights right away about discipline issues," explained Alan during a particularly difficult session. "I saw the not-so-nice side of my bride pretty quickly," he finished with a bit of a smile.

Family System Issues

The honeymoon can dissipate relatively quickly, given the reality of how difficult the stepmother role really is. Regardless of whether she brings her own biological or adopted children into the new family, there are still "wicked stepmother" myths. Nonetheless, she has to acquaint herself with and blend with her partner's children. Furthermore, in our culture it is still usually expected that the woman will be responsible for the emotional life of the family. It is particularly difficult, then, for a woman to have the parenting responsibility for stepchildren who challenge her authority and her love. She wants nothing more than to parent, yet this is denied her. Meanwhile, she may fight with the man she loves, whom she wants to father her child, merely because his children represent a history she didn't share and won't ever fully belong to.

In the nuclear family into which a child is born or adopted, the couple's focus and energy shifts from the marital dyad to the family triad. This shift generates significant issues regarding their relationship to one another as well as their relationships to their child: They have to negotiate a new balance and new alliances within the triangular configuration. Similarly, the stepfamily attempts to deal with the numerous triangular relationships of parents, stepparents, and children by juggling alliances. It is not uncommon for a new stepfamily to attempt to manage conflict by placing the issues in the parent-child system even if they belong in the couple system. The fear of another marital breakup makes it less threatening for the couple to place the blame on the stepparent-child relationship.

The gender balance is changed so there are issues around gender as well as issues around inclusion or exclusion. The degree of attachment the mother feels toward the child may set off issues within the whole system around autonomy or dependence and separation or loss. Such issues can be magnified if the couple has also experienced the losses associated with infertility or an unsuccessful adoption attempt. Likewise, stepfamilies wrestle with issues of inclusion and exclusion, but the configuration includes more players since there exist other parents who usually remain actively involved. When the stepfamily is comprised of a single adoptive parent marrying a divorced parent there is a convergence of still more levels of loss and attachment, autonomy and dependence.

Balancing Parent and Partner Roles

Parents in these variant family configurations struggle with numerous developmental issues that transcend both the individual and the couple system. They struggle with where they fit or how to fit, where they are wanted and included. At the same time, they struggle with the intense feelings in their hearts. As Alan said, "I love Joy very much and I want her to be happy. I also love my children very much. I think I understand how painful her emptiness is and how badly she desires another child. That only increases my pain. We have become so absorbed in this struggle that it has hurt our relationship. We still have to parent these kids when they visit—and frequently over the phone—but for now I want my wife back."

Joy is aware of the burden her unhappiness has placed on Alan and on their relationship; however, she also suffers with a heavy heart. In the early stages of their marriage, when Alan and his children filled so much of her life, she could never have anticipated the emptiness she would now feel. She could not have anticipated what this childlessness would feel like, nor how empty it would feel even with Alan by her side. The parent and the partner roles had unwittingly become so integrated that she now feels a tremendous vacuum created by the loss of Alan's children in her daily routines.

Implications for Therapy

Variant family forms produce their own sets of problems and issues. Sometimes couples, like Alan and Joy, enter therapy in order to have a safe arena in which to discuss parenting issues. Other couples or individuals enter therapy to discuss their desire to become parents and whether this is a viable option for them. Many of their issues will be similar regardless of whether they constitute a heterosexual or gay or lesbian couple, a stepfamily, or a single individual. Some of the more general issues include:

- Exploring the various reproductive or adoptive options.
- Discussing specifically what each option entails: It helps clients to have some sense of what to expect—medically and psychologically—from the various options and treatments.
- Helping them gain a sense of the time, energy, and financial investment required: This helps them determine what is viable for them, given their lifestyle and resources.

Specific Issues

Singles and gay and lesbian couples need to explore the complicated issues related to donor inseminations. They must review the positive and negative consequences of a known versus unknown donor in order to understand the psychological and legal ramifications. Lesbian and gay couples may have to struggle with issues surrounding coming out if they have not previously. Lesbian couples also have to struggle with the decision about which partner will become pregnant and how the birth certificate will read.

Out-of-phase couples must examine significant lifestyle issues. If one partner has brought children into the stepfamily, how will additional children impact the situation? If there are no children, how will having a child this late in life affect their lifestyle?

In addition to helping these singles, gay or lesbian couples, or out-of-phase couples address the many general and specific issues they need to confront, the therapist must also help them work through many of the stages infertile individuals have to face. They have experienced a crisis, one that will affect them and all of their relationships, albeit to different degrees, forever. They have experienced tremendous disappointment and loss. Loss of dreams, self-esteem, and perhaps a family as they fantasized it. They will feel angry and resentful, just as infertile individuals do, toward others who have children easily, those who mistreat children, and perhaps toward partners who have delayed or inhibited their ability to have children. They must struggle to articulate these feelings and then to work through such strong feelings.

Many who are involuntarily childless will also feel guilty about past behaviors, particularly sexual behaviors. However, they may also feel guilty around life decisions which they believe they should have rendered differently. A man may wish he had married his college sweetheart and not postponed marriage. A lesbian may wish she had come out sooner to her family so she and her lesbian partner could have tried to adopt her friend's child when he became available for adoption. Perhaps another woman feels she should have married and started a family before entering law school. Even though the involuntarily childless may feel varying levels of resentment, anger, or guilt, they all experience raised levels of depression. They are depressed regarding what hasn't been and what might never be. They are depressed because, like those who are infertile, they feel helpless. So much of what they are experiencing is beyond their control, even though it is not attributable to infertility. They must recognize and then work through these feelings piece by piece. They must find resolution, whether that involves making peace with a nonbiological or stepchild or child-free living. They must let go of the past and make the future into something that has meaning for them.

COMMITMENT TO PARENTHOOD

Everyone has concerns about the commitment of parenthood, so encouraging the expression of such uncertainties will create relief and perhaps allow the issue to be more thoroughly addressed. Particularly for singles considering parenthood, attention should be directed toward examining the reality of their life demands in conjunction with the demands they are facing as a single parent.

It is useful to help clients assess their available social and familial supports. Some of this exploration may encompass examination of religious and cultural issues. Religious and cultural factors can be a source of comfort and support for these individuals during future challenges. (For a more thorough discussion of the impact of cultural and religious factors see chapter 5.) However, single parents especially need more than social or emotional support. They need practical support, like good childcare, emergency backup, a ride to the hospital or other appointments, and some opportunities for just relaxing. The following dialogue with Linda, the 32-year-old teacher, illustrates the importance of helping the client assess such support.

Linda: You know my parents and my sister live nearby. I know they will be a great support for me, and even though my sister has two kids I know she'd take mine too in a pinch.

Therapist: Linda, it isn't merely a matter of childcare; it's about "Linda care" too. You will need some time out. You want a social life, you have doctor and dentist appointments and haircuts and so on. You need to be thinking of how you will accommodate these realities.

Linda: I know. But I just can't imagine that I'll want to be away from my child much at all—after all I've gone through to have one. But if, as you say, I need to consider these realities, I will. I'm thinking of having a part-time nanny; I would think that would be quite sufficient.

Therapist: I know you're getting a little irritated with all of these issues, Linda. And I know how badly you want this child and that you have already jumped over numerous hurdles in order to receive the donor inseminations. I just want you to be clear about the intense level of commitment you are signing up for. You essentially will have two full-time careers, between your teaching and carrying the full load for this child, as the only parent.

Although most single parents indicate that their mother and sisters are their first sources of support and friends are a good second source, most have a difficult time asking for help. Because they have usually been independent, goal-oriented, and professionally successful, they are surprised that they even need help. Single parents must understand that there will be times when they are anxious or sick or otherwise need assistance. They actually need to learn to ask for help and to understand that doing so is not an indication of failure or weakness—it is a natural part of the single parent experience. In fact, according to Melina (1986), single adoptive parents who were able to ask for assistance believed their adjustment period went more smoothly and attachment developed more quickly because they had good support from friends and relatives.

Whether an adoptive or biological parent, single or couple, support groups can also be quite helpful. Since many decide to become parents despite obstacles or resistance, they often feel the need to be superparents. They often have difficulty acknowledging their feelings of discontent, inadequacy or sense of failure. It is consequential then for these parents to hear others struggling with the same frustrations or issues and to be able to glean ideas to help them cope and feel some support around their own issues. "I feel such relief," explained Marie, the 34-year-old nail technician. "It is so good to hear that other single parents sometimes feel resentful. After hearing other mothers talk about feeling weird when people ask about the baby's dad, I don't feel so alone or weird. I really look forward to the group too; it's almost a social time, and I have become friendly with two of the other members."

ADOPTION ISSUES

Single parents of adoptive children, whether never married or divorced, need assistance addressing issues specific to the adoptive process. For example, when they come for therapy with parent-child difficulties it is important to determine whether the problems seem to be part of the parent-child relationship or merely transition issues. There are transition issues in biologically-based families and stepfamilies also, but the transitions are not complicated by the many losses or unknowns encountered in the adoptive situation. When an adoption is open, a more popular and recommended alternative today, the adoptive parents and the birthparent(s) know about one another, including details about each other's lives; sometimes they have met. They often work out, through the social service agency or adoption lawyer, parameters for contact. Thus, the role of the birthparents can be either a stressor or a positive factor for both the adoptee and his or her adopting parents. Often, the actual encounter with the birthparents is not what was fantasized: The adoptive parents may have had fantasies about somehow coparenting this child and thus when the birthparent(s) falter, they too experience disillusionment, betrayal, and abandonment.

The life stage of each family member is another significant issue for therapy with adoptive parents. An older parent adopting an adolescent can exacerbate numerous mid-life issues for the parent. Likewise, the adolescent who is struggling to form her sexuality and identity will have many biases about an older-appearing parent. This may constitute another type of loss for the adoptive child. She may feel she has lost her fantasized parent as well as her birthparent(s). The therapeutic setting then offers a safe, neutral forum in which the single adoptive parent and the adoptee can articulate these fears, frustrations, and losses.

DONOR INSEMINATION ISSUES

The donor procedure, whether involving a known or anonymous donor, raises significant questions for singles or parents opting for this procedure. Singles have to look at the issue of not having an identified or available father in the picture. Although this may be the desired goal and thus not a problem, it nonetheless needs to be directly addressed.

One of the most central and difficult questions, of course, is whether to disclose to others, especially the child, the method of conception. Lesbian couples and single women are more likely to disclose to numerous others and to tell the child (Jacob, in press). It is understandable that they feel more disposed toward disclosure since it is more apparent; a single woman or two women in a relationship would not likely become accidentally pregnant. Heterosexual couples can more easily hide the fact of donor insemination and thus may be less likely to disclose to others. "Before we conceived, we knew that we would tell our child how very much we wanted her and exactly how she was conceived," commented Melissa, the 36-year-old physician. "I find it so interesting that my cousin and his wife received donor inseminations and don't want to tell the child or anyone else. I think their doctors even support their secrecy. Of course it was a lot simpler for them because they're heterosexual. It sure stands out a lot more when an unmarried female—lesbian or not—becomes pregnant."

The issue becomes more complicated upon closer examination. It may be simple to decide not to tell friends or even family, but if there are school problems, should the teacher or school psychologist be apprised? What if there are medical problems? Should the pediatrician be advised? If the single or couple presents for therapy prior to the decision about becoming parents, or prior to the insemination, all of these issues can be addressed. Once they become parents the issues can still be addressed, but the context becomes more emotional, perhaps more threatening—and certainly more complex.

Even though many physicians still encourage secrecy, the dynamics created by keeping a secret in the family set up unhealthy balances in the family system. The secret becomes triangulated into the family dynamics, creating a powerful specter that is never directly talked about or resolved. Additionally, while such secrecy may serve to protect a child's privacy, it will also keep secret any significant information about her biological father. Although it is never suggested that a couple include their child in their private affairs, it may be useful for the child to be aware of this particular struggle, of how important his or her existence has been to them.

Special Issues for Gay and Lesbian Couples

The questions about whether and whom to tell about the donor procedure involve whether to tell the child. This query becomes real and public with the decision about what to put on the birth certificate. Of course, this also involves decisions about whether to attempt to place both parents' names on the birth certificate. If the gay or lesbian couple have not yet struggled with the issues around coming out to their own families, it would be appropriate to address this in the therapy at this time. They need to confront the issues that surround becoming a more formalized family and the ramifications of disclosure—or not—for the members of this family. Thus, they need to struggle not only with disclosure of the donor insemination procedure, but also of their gay or lesbian lifestyle. Completing the coming-out process can be an important step in preparation for the donor insemination procedure so the child will not have to bear the burden of such secrets. "Sandy and I didn't have any disagreement about whether to tell our child about the donor inseminations," explained Melissa. "We *do* have a problem regarding how to deal with Sandy's parents. I think all of these decisions and procedures create an opportune time for Sandy to finally come out with them. I mean, after all, her 'roommate' is going be pregnant and then have this baby that Sandy is going to dote over. So I think it will start to look suspicious. I would like to resolve our level of openness more clearly now—especially with her parents."

Using therapy to examine and struggle with the issues of family formation are just as essential with gay or lesbian couples as with heterosexual couples. In fact, it is important to recognize that "the therapist working with a same-sex couple should not make the naive assumption that, because this couple is not infertile, decisions about whether and how to become parents together will not be problematic" (Brown, 1995, p. 288). The decision process is similar in many ways to that of a heterosexual couple, but may involve these other disclosure issues, depending upon how the couple has dealt with issues thus far. Just as in a heterosexual relationship, the frustration in not being able to easily fulfill a life goal aggravates other problems in the relationship.

In addition, gay and lesbian couples have to plan more carefully if they want children—even if they are not infertile it is, of course, more complicated for them to become pregnant. "I just assumed I'd never have the opportunity to be a mom," explained Melissa in an early session. "Then, one day I realized that just because I'm a lesbian doesn't mean I can't be a mom. I started reading some information about inseminations and realized I could get pregnant even without a man in my life and even though I'm not heterosexual." Melissa had dealt with her ambivalence about her sexual orientation. She was now beginning to explore her reasons for wanting to be a mother and establishing the emotional and practical supports for that possibility. Her self-esteem began to improve as she realized she could make this dream happen and work for her and her partner. They had already dealt with the next step, the decision about who would carry the pregnancy, a decision that for many couples is a significant stumbling block during therapy. The inseminations place a monthly strain on the relationship; these couples experience the same roller coaster of emotions as infertile couples. In addition, the co-mother may experience feelings of envy or of being left out during the course of the inseminations. This can become exacerbated with the advent of a pregnancy as the pregnant partner becomes more preoccupied with her body. The partner may feel that the desired child is more important than she is and begin to feel the power imbalance. Of course, these are common feelings in heterosexual relationships and it helps the lesbian couple to have such feelings normalized.

The feelings of being left out and the sense of loss that accompanies all of these occurrences continue to escalate when the child is born and as she grows. Because she has no legal standing with respect to the child, the co-mother feels invisible with the significant players in her child's life. It is apparent, then, how important the initial therapy sessions must be in assisting these couples to resolve their relationship and co-mother issues, address parenting and discipline issues, and learn healthy conflict resolution and communication skills. Melissa and Sandy worked quite hard to address their conflicts.

Sandy: It was so important to me when you insisted last session that Melissa and I must present a united front with our discipline. I feel that since she will carry our child, she has more entitlement in most areas of our child's life.

Melissa: And I have told you many times not to feel that way! You are backing off from so many decisions because of this thing you have about entitlement and who will be pregnant. Pregnancy is only one small aspect of parenthood.

Therapist: That's a good point, Melissa, and an important one. You two are allowing the pregnancy and child to come between you. You have lost some of the ability to communicate about your relationship, your fears, and your desires. You both told me that had always been an important aspect of your relationship, one of the things that had always made it so special. I know this is a complicated and emotion-laden issue, but don't let go of those important relationship strengths now.

Considerations for Out-of-Phase Couples

Melanie and Rick, who were introduced on page 134, must deal with issues that are typical of out-of-phase couples. "My loss is just as real as my cousin's," cried Melanie during one emotional session. "Just because I'm not infertile doesn't mean I'm not just as upset about not being pregnant and not having a child." Melanie was finally able to express her anger toward Rick. She talked about feeling betrayed and resentful because he didn't want to have children. Rick, too, felt angry, because he believed Melanie had retracted their original marital agreement about a child-free marriage, even though it had never been a formalized agreement. Therapy with these couples is similar to that with infertile couples. The therapist can help the spouses do several things:

- Express their anger.
- Face conflicts head on, listen to one another without becoming defensive or thinking they have to make their case.
- Examine the meaning of children in their lives at this point in time.
- Set some mutually satisfying goals for their marriage and their lives together.
- Examine their individual goals and values.
- Finally, they may need to question whether the marriage is a healthy and satisfying one and then take appropriate steps to improve their situation.

Although many of the issues addressed in therapy are specific to singles, gay and lesbian couples, or out-of-phase couples, other issues are shared by all individuals struggling with the enormous life issues of children and parenting. All individuals, regardless of their developmental stage, feel the magnitude of the decision to parent or not. What few comprehend initially is the strain they may encounter when life does not continue in a predictable and controllable path.

8

THE IMPLICATIONS OF
BIOTECHNOLOGY FOR THE
FAMILY AND THE CULTURE

THE HIGH-TECH SOLUTIONS employed to help the involuntarily childless become parents have created a variety of family forms that confound our conventional knowledge and usual assumptions. Our current definitions of family have become restrictive because they do not take into account the personal, political, and social consequences of what has become possible through the biotechnical revolution.

Traditionally, parenthood was believed to begin with the birth of one's biologically-related progeny. Throughout history the genetic link has defined family boundaries, duties, and obligations (Jaeger, 1996). The separation of genetics from gestation was unimaginable and unthinkable since family was primarily defined by bloodlines, with the exception of adoptive family configurations. All cultures held strongly established values around reproduction and the acceptance of a new member into the community.

Only decades ago reproductive medicine focused on preventing pregnancy; today the emphasis is on creating life. This change of focus has precipitated concern that the new technology has started us on a course with enormous consequences for the children who are created, the traditional family, and society as a whole. "As medical and scientific progress changes the way in which people can become a family and have a family, it has caused changes that stretch the traditional concept of genetic ties defining family structure" (Jaeger, 1996, p. 113).

The mere existence of third-party gamete donors has forced a differentiation between biological, gestational, and social mother. With the advent of reliable birth control, sex without reproduction has challenged the concept of parenting and family formation as the epitome of life's goals. Today, reproduction without sex further jolts our sense of conventional societal values and the very foundation of the traditional family (Herz, 1989).

Variant family forms created by the permutations and combinations possible with biotechnology force reconsideration of our definitions of family. Family-building arrangements, which were historically clandestine, are presently the topics of the scientific, theological, and legal discussions. Understandably, advanced biotechnical procedures challenge conventional societal standards. Social, psychological, and ethical issues raised by these procedures provoke considerable discussion and confusion. Legal and social definitions of parenthood now lag behind the medical technology that makes parenthood possible.

In the United States, decisions about whether and when to have children are considered to be matters of personal concern and not subject to government interference. Individuals' rights regarding reproductive choice are protected. However, due to such complex medical processes as gamete donation and gestational surrogacy, a child may have as many as five parents. So, as biological and legal parentage become distinct, the legal system is called upon to mediate the respective rights and duties of the many parties involved. New schemas and new policies are needed in order to create a secure and growth-enhancing environment for these children and the variant families being formed. Nuclear and extended families must find new ways of relating and novel ways of defining family in order to support the new family configuration.

Redefining the Family

Involuntarily childless and infertile singles and couples are living in a unique era of history. The technological explosion of new methods for achieving pregnancy provides a new lens through which to view typical family-building and the traditional family. New family configurations and dynamics are created not only by married heterosexual couples, but also by single men and women and gay and lesbian couples. For instance, when a gay couple decides to have a child through a surrogate, the family has been redefined: it is no longer the traditional male-female two-parent family. Half of the child's biology is connected with a woman he may never again have contact with, or who may be peripheral in his life. "I'm happy with my family," explained 9-year-old Tom one day. "It's just so different. Even though I live with two parents who act just like my friend's parents, with rules and all that stuff, I go to the park or to gymnastics with two guys. All of my friends ask their moms if they can go out; I have to ask my two dads. It's weird. I don't even know what my mom—my biological mom— really looks like."

The traditional male-female two parent family is also redefined when a child is conceived through donor insemination. Gerald and Alice came into therapy shortly after their daughter was born. "Melissa was conceived through donor sperm," explained Gerald, a computer analyst. "We decided we want to tell her about, you know, this donor. We just aren't sure how or when. How do we address this other person? We believe that we are Melissa's family, but we feel like the donor's here somehow too. I can't just erase him even if I wanted to. And yet she'll never know him. He wants his privacy even though he's such an integral part of our family."

Even though kinship relationships have traditionally been based on connections among persons tied by blood or marriage, today we are aware that we do not need blood or biology to create strong, loving relationships among adults and children. The key ingredients are mutual caring and a strong bond.

Oocyte donation, a newer development, creates questions about the mother, about who she might really be. Prior to advanced reproductive techniques, the definition of "mother" was simple. She was the one who raised the children. Now the rearing mother may not be the biological mother, and she may not even have carried the pregnancy. If we also add in the two possible roles a father could contribute, the biological and the rearing father, a child could ostensibly have as many as five contributors to parental roles.

Donor sperm and surrogacy are not new concepts. Third-party involvement with donor sperm has been practiced since Biblical times. Sarah directed Abraham to have a child with her maid, but expected that she and Abraham would raise the child. What is new and different is the degree of technology involved with reproduction and the fact that oftentimes this technology offers highly sophisticated means for reproduction. This creates a dilemma when the parent(s) and families are forced to examine the implications and consequences of all that comes along with the technology. Vera and Steve are very grateful to be parents of a little boy. However, "we never could have anticipated all of the complex issues we're having to face," explained Vera, a 43-year-old organizational consultant. "I don't know what or when to tell Jacob about his biological mother. Steve isn't sure he wants to tell him much at all. I feel funny telling him his gestational mom, the one who carried him, answered an ad we placed, and just seemed like the right person. It all just seems so strange." Steve, a 45-year-old carpenter added, "I just want him to feel loved and normal. I don't want to make a big deal out of all this, but I don't want to live with secrets either, as if we're ashamed of anything."

"Although the forms of the family have changed, people are still trying to fit the new, sometimes called 'alternative,' family into the traditional model of the two-parent nuclear family as the only 'right' kind of family" (Biddle, Roszia, & Silverstein, 1995, p. 17). To force these new family systems into the old assumptions inherent in the two-parent biological family can create a sense of isolation, identity confusion, and alienation. Often these families feel as though they are drifting in uncharted waters, not knowing where to look for definition or direction. "There were no books on these issues when we started—not that we knew where to look or even looked very hard. We were too busy focusing on just becoming parents," Vera continued to explain. "We didn't know who to talk to. Of course we didn't know other couples who were going through donor programs and there weren't many who had gone before us to give us a sense of what they experienced—and they weren't going public 15 years ago." Steve added, "The support group that we found about eight years ago has been quite helpful in terms of support, but no one seems to have any great answers about how, when, or what to tell these kids. There is no Dr.

Spock to turn to about these issues, and there isn't any long-term psychological research to depend on yet either."

New technology requires innovative ways of looking at the configurations created and examining the long- and short-term implications. We need new paradigms, creative ways of looking at these new family forms. It is conceivable that the new families will be stronger and more resilient because of the high level of commitment needed to get through the rigors of such treatments. Nonetheless, they require new models of support and kinship to accommodate their unique family system. The very strengths that assisted them to come into being should be harnessed to empower them.

Moral and Ethical Issues

Reproductive technology has developed at such a rapid rate that our culture has not kept pace with its moral and ethical implications. As with any new medical advance, there are troubling ethical questions regarding whether we really *should* do what we are now *able* to do (Mahowald, 1996). It is difficult to anticipate the long-range implications of current reproductive options.

As is true of all progress, the picture is not always positive or clear for individuals or society as a whole. Many express ambivalence about the complexity of the technology, the enormous commitment of time, energy, and financial resources, and the ethical aspects of the assisted reproduction methods. Some worry about manipulating nature, forgetting that medical science is about intercepting nature's course. Many are concerned that creating life outside of the body may denigrate the reverence for human life, or may even create some kind of monster. Many have reservations regarding ethical and moral considerations with respect to gay and lesbian parents even though these variant families are functioning in healthy ways and raising adaptive children.

For the infertile or involuntarily childless, the options are not without problems. The many options and accompanying weighty considerations contribute to the emotional distress these individuals experience. Nonetheless, in a follow-up study of couples after unsuccessful in vitro fertilization, Leiblum (1988) reported that 93 percent said that if another reproductive option for a biological child came along, they would elect such a procedure. Such determination is remarkable in light of the adoption alternative; most individuals still place a premium on a biological or genetic connection with their wished-for children. This biological connection may be one of the primary reasons that donor insemination is a widely sought treatment.

Others may experience the new technology as a more significant dilemma and added pressure. "Some feminists believe that the quest for new reproductive options reinforces the notion that the only acceptable role for women is motherhood and that women who voluntarily opt for child-free lives are either selfish or deficient in their womanhood" (Leiblum, 1988, p. 132). Men and women, whether single, gay, lesbian, or heterosexual, have come to believe that reproduction is a God-given right. They feel they are entitled to all available technological options.

But when these individuals become parents and have to face their children and the ramifications of their actions, they are confronted with questions and concerns that are larger than they could have imagined. "Ironically, the process of using new technology to produce children has created embryonic orphans" (Holbrook, 1990, p. 336). Trying to explain or rationalize reproductive decisions has proven more complex and emotionally intense than any parent could have anticipated.

"We wanted a child so badly," explained Karen, a 48-year-old bank teller. "We just didn't think. We didn't really think about what Emily would say when we told her about donor sperm, that her biological dad was known only as a test tube. I never knew how much pain she would now feel that she can never see him, ask him questions, or learn about his family." Dan, Emily's rearing father, expressed his concerns too: "I sometimes feel she's mad at me or disappointed in me because I'm not her biological father. I wonder if she feels betrayed somehow."

The Role of Religion

In times of such uncertainty and inner turmoil, many turn to their religion (see chapter 5). However, the assisted reproductive technologies also represent religious dilemmas. Throughout history there has been an emphasis on continuity of the culture. This has been ensured through family and religious and cultural rituals that celebrate fertility and reproduction. As a result, rules around reproductive behavior are some of the most rigidly held and fiercely defended values in all cultures.

Some clergy believe the techniques symbolize a manipulation of human life and are therefore unacceptable on religious grounds. For example, donor insemination and in vitro fertilization are controversial among religious leaders because singles, gays, and lesbians may be inseminated as well as heterosexual married couples. A new life is created outside of the "normal" method of sexual intercourse, a practice some religious leaders perceive as wrong and therefore unacceptable.

There have been religious and ethical concerns about in vitro fertilization since the birth of Louise Brown in 1978. Many consider the "test tube baby" unnatural and a violation of the natural order. Critics argue that the "separation of lovemaking from life giving [is] bound to lead to a degradation of the marital covenant with dire consequences for the child, the traditional institution of the family, and hence for society as a whole" (Herz, 1989, p. 119). Advocates of the IVF procedure argue that there now exists a way in which human creativity can assist what nature has difficulty producing. Proponents also argue that the sanctity of human life is more dependent on an attitude of respect than the specific location of fertilization.

Secrecy

Donor insemination entails numerous layers of psychological distress. The secrecy component and the struggle surrounding whether to disclose the secret contribute to immense levels of stress and can interfere with the couple's intimacy. So, even though the couple may believe they have moved beyond their infertility, the family dynamics may be disrupted. Those who proceed with donor insemination confront numerous psychological and ethical issues throughout the child's development.

Even though some men may find it easier to accept the child when the origins remain secret, concerns about the potential psychological impact on the child arise (Herz, 1989). If the child is not told about the infertility or donor insemination, she is unknowingly deprived of the basic facts about her very origin. Secrecy can become counterproductive if the child desires to trace genetic diseases or other family traits or even the family history of the biological father. In 1983, Phil Donahue interviewed young women in their twenties who were conceived by donor insemination. These women expressed anger about the destruction of the medical records. They desired more information about their biological fathers, especially medical information (Mechaneck et al., 1988). It is unknown whether these women would push to obtain other types of information given the opportunity, but it is important to note the intensity of their feelings regarding these issues. (Many adoptees have similar feelings of curiosity or anger about their biological parents. A significant difference, however, is that most adult adoptees have access to their biological mothers and can therefore access information about their biological fathers even if they never have access to him directly.)

Interestingly, even though single women take longer than marrieds to decide to proceed with donor insemination, they are more likely to tell the child about his or her origins (Jacob, in press). This may be connected to the fact that these children become aware that there is no apparent male or father figure in the picture and ultimately question their origins more readily than children of marrieds. Although married couples are more able to protect this intimate aspect of their lives, it does not make secrecy any less dysfunctional for this child or the partners.

When medical personnel encourage the secrecy or agree to maintain a secret, thus colluding with one or both partners, they become part of a larger dilemma: the question about whether to disclose or not. Until there is more information regarding the effects of disclosure, or lack of it, they could be engaging in ethically questionable behavior. Although women who choose not to disclose usually do so to protect their partner's image, his potency or masculinity, the basis for such a decision raises ethical issues regarding conflicting interests of the parents and child (Herz, 1989). At the very least these children deserve access to records of their biological father's medical and genetic history. A system should be in place to alert the child and/or family if the health of the donor changes in unanticipated ways.

Considerations for Reproductive Programs

PATIENT SCREENING

Although medical personnel may be comfortable with the IVF procedure as a medical process, they may not necessarily be comfortable with the implications of treating alternative couples or singles. Often the reproductive staff feel some responsibility for a child born because of their assistance and thus believe they have a significant level of ethical obligation. Such a sense of obligation can set up an evaluation process to assess an individual's or couple's competence for parenthood prior to performing the IVF treatments. It is not that they are attempting to be religious or moral gatekeepers, but rather that as assistants in creating life in circumstances that are atypical, they work to insure they are performing a service for responsible, functional people.

SURROGACY

Surrogate parenting is opposed by many on moral grounds on the premise that it involves third-party baby-selling (Salzer, 1991). Many clergy and others in society have difficulty with the concept of a woman gestating a child for the exchange of money. Holbrook (1990) fears that "fees for surrogacy could result in an underclass of breeder women" (Holbrook, p. 335), perhaps evoking visions of *1984* or *Brave New World*. On the other hand, those who support paid surrogacy argue that surrogate mothers are not paid for the baby, but rather for the time, effort, and pain of bearing the child. The process of gestating and giving birth raises important questions about balancing the autonomy and well-being of the surrogate while she is gestating a child for another to rear (Jaeger, 1996). Financial remuneration is certainly a form of compensation that may offset any discomfort or pain the surrogate experiences.

Interestingly, however, most of the women who become surrogates indicate that their primary reason was in fact altruistic. They welcome the opportunity to help an infertile couple, although sometimes the surrogacy experience is sought as a way to relieve unresolved guilt from a previous abortion or prior promiscuity (Herz, 1989).

Most of what has been written about surrogacy has focused on the rights, obligations, and responsibilities of the parents (Parker, 1983, 1984; Robertson, 1983). Ethically, we need to also consider the implications of surrogacy for the child involved. As in the case of donor insemination, what or how much should the child be told? What happens in a case where the child is malformed and neither the contracting parents nor the surrogate want the child (Herz, 1989)?

EGG AND EMBRYO DONATION

A reproductive option closely related to donor insemination is egg donation. With these procedures, the resulting child has the genetic make-up of at least one parent. Many of the same issues confront these parents regarding the effects on the donor, the family, and most significantly, the child. Sometimes when the egg donor is known, or is a family member, she may feel she has the right to intervene in the family dynamics or with the child. Again, technology has surpassed psychology's knowledge regarding how to support and counsel these new family systems and the multitude of players.

With cryopreservation technology, embryos can be frozen and donated. Children created from these embryos have no lineal genetic relation to their rearing parents. These children are different from adopted children because adopted children are already in existence when rearing parents are sought. Another, probably unanticipated, dilemma with cryopreserved embryos is that they could skip one or more generations before they are used. In the future this could lead to a disruption of family or societal structures. Since the culture is having difficulty keeping pace with the technology, it is not clear how accurately or in what detail the records are kept during the cryopreservation.

The ethical and moral issues needing consideration transcend the technology of the reproductive procedures. The variant family forms which result create even larger cultural issues. The very purpose and definition of the family in this new cultural context need to be examined. What might be the consequences of single parenthood on the psychological development of the child? How will this affect the child's ability to form relationships with the opposite sex? More longitudinal research is called for in order to begin to address such momentous issues because they have significant implications for the continued use of the biotechnology and its societal impact.

Often moral issues and policy issues are accompanied by legal issues. As the legal system struggles to define rights and ownership, medical and research personnel struggle over the social and moral decisions regarding disposition of donated eggs and cryopreserved embryos. As is true with many medical decisions, values become commingled with other issues. Who will make the decision regarding whether postmenopausal women can receive donated eggs? Should research interests have priority over singles or couples who wish the donated eggs? These are ethical, moral, and legal questions which may require more complex responses than we have been prepared to accommodate.

SOCIOECONOMIC CONSIDERATIONS

There are also socioeconomic discrepancies which need to be addressed. Infertility affects all people regardless of financial status, but because the poor do not have equal access to medical care, they may not have equal access to infertility treatment. Such discrepancies are unjust and reflect negatively on our culture and its values. How this will affect the culture in the future remains to be seen. It will be difficult to build on a structure that is flawed with inequity, where all children and even wished-for children do not have equal opportunities.

Societal Responses

There have been some attempts to address such inequities and to address other ethical issues presented by biotechnology. As a result of the Helsinki Declaration, institutional review boards were developed in the 1960s to review ethical issues around proposals for biomedical research (Hindle, 1996). The focus of the boards is to review biomedical research to ensure the rights of human subjects and to deal with the ethical issues the research presented. The boards are regulated by federal and state governments, who define the composition of the board and its activities. Such boards help to emphasize the emerging need for regulation and vigilance. Even though they were set up to address only issues surrounding research, the presence of the boards helped germinate the idea of regulating the techniques themselves.

The next step was the creation of bioethics committees. These committees deal with the moral and ethical dilemmas arising from the use of the already established techniques, rather than merely focusing on the developing techniques, which is the emphasis of the review boards. Such committees, often located in hospitals, include case review and serve a supportive, consultative role to medical personnel. Often the committee will address issues such as quality of life or the right to refuse treatment and will make recommendations to the hospital board regarding education and policy development. The committee has become a significant avenue for discourse about these weighty issues. It is a necessary but not sufficient step in dealing with the ramifications of biotechnical advancement.

A further responsible step was taken by the medical community. The American Society of Reproductive Medicine convened the Council on Ethical and Judicial Affairs (CEJA) and the Council on Scientific Affairs (CSA) in December 1995. The Councils are comprised of representatives from specialty societies and federal agencies. They are concerned about the practice of ART and were formed to respond to occasions of abuse and unethical conduct. The representatives emphasize the need for monitoring their work: "Given the rapid technological progress and unique profit motive in ART, reinforcing ethical guidelines is especially vital" (Plows & Howe, 1996, p. 2). The report issues specific recommendations for medical personnel and labs, and for potential legislative action. They address issues such as honesty in advertising ART services, integrity in terms of informing patients regarding risks and benefits, and standardizing consent forms for patients. Not only must the benefits of ART be disclosed to patients, but the limitations or risks as well. Certainly the report provides a most significant beginning because it creates guidelines while also giving a meaningful message about the importance of regulation. However, it is material to bear in mind that traditional bioethical guidelines may not be sufficient to deal with the sophisticated ethical, legal, and social implications the technology will render.

Legal Issues

Our society does not regulate conception. The constitutional right to privacy protects reproductive decisions and gives clear precedence to the autonomy of the couple over government or state regulations (Herz, 1989; Jaeger, 1996). Many become parents and repeat the process as often as they choose even if they are unfit for the job. The law will only intervene after birth if the child's welfare is considered to be at risk. Arguably then, just because the means of conception have changed, neither society, the legal system, nor a physician should have the right to regulate who should become parents. In fact, the law now protects the right to reproduce noncoitally through the judgment rendered in the Baby M case (Jaeger, 1996).

The Baby M case (*In re Baby M*, 1988) is a well-known New Jersey custody case of a child conceived by artificial insemination of a surrogate mother. After the birth, the surrogate mother decided she could not relinquish the child. The New Jersey Supreme Court held that the man providing the sperm was the legal father and the woman providing the egg and carrying the pregnancy—not the woman who contracted the surrogate—was the legal mother (*In re Baby M*, 1988). The court ultimately awarded custody to the genetic father and his spouse, but granted visitation rights to the surrogate. Although the case focused on the surrogate contract, the court also addressed the constitutional right of privacy. The court asserted that the constitutional right of privacy protects the decision to reproduce coitally; that right also extends to decisions to reproduce noncoitally (Jaeger, 1996).

In any society, social attitudes often become confused with individuals' rights. However, social disapproval of nontraditional families does not constitute a compelling reason to withhold reproductive measures. Fortunately, as the legal system has been challenged, protection of reproductive decisions has been extended to individuals as well as married couples.

As these issues continue to challenge society and the legal system, "it will often be critical to make distinctions, usually previously irrelevant, between the genetic, gestational, and rearing parents when sorting out individual rights and responsibilities" (Annas & Elias, 1989, p. 614). One factor that may assist in the distinction, at least in a moral sense, would be examination of intention (Mahowald, 1996). Sperm, egg, and embryo donors do not intend to be rearing parents. But if the intention of these donors shifts, there should be legal provisions for distinguishing parental rights and responsibilities.

Donor Insemination

Legal parameters are needed to mediate the unique relationships being generated by the biotechnical procedures. The courts need to expand the very definition of family beyond those who are biologically or maritally related or adopted. The problem lies in finding ways to construct consistent, even-handed laws that are fair to all parties. For example, with donor inseminations, a donor requests anonymity and prefers waiving his rights to any resulting children. Many states have passed laws designating the consenting husband as the legal father of the offspring. The donor, however, may be better protected with a contract rather than a consent form since he is really merely a "sperm vendor" (Annas & Elias, 1989). In a similar situation, a sperm donor to a surrogate certainly may wish to retain all rights to a resulting child and thus must be carefully distinguished from the previous category of sperm donor.

Surrogacy also brings up issues of commercialization of motherhood, which many believe needs regulation. For example, among numerous issues that can create a legal morass with surrogacy, a surrogate can change her mind and refuse to relinquish the child and sue the donor for child support. Even though the legal system maintains that sperm donors and surrogates have signed away their rights prior to birth, every time a case is brought before the courts the legal system is again forced to grapple with what constitutes a family. In vitro fertilization forces examination of the issues around who may become a candidate for the procedure. The medical community has had to face the dilemma of whether to limit the procedure to married couples, or just to couples, even if of the same sex, without benefit of legal guidelines.

Despite the ethical or moral reservations, what has remained of utmost importance within the legal community has been safeguarding an individual's right to reproductive autonomy. Therefore, focus has been directed toward regulating the procedures rather than regulating the legality of donor inseminations or who may become a donor recipient. For example, with donor sperm some steps have been made toward uniform standards for screening the applicants beyond screening just for medical and health issues. It has also been suggested that the number of offspring per donor be limited or monitored nationally (Herz, 1989; Pakizegi, 1990) so that incidents such as that occurring with Dr. Cecil Jacobson do not again take place. Dr. Jacobson was convicted in 1992 of fraud and perjury after federal prosecutors charged he fathered as many as 75 children through donor insemination with his own sperm and misrepresented to his patients information about the true donor (*United States v. Jacobson,* 1992). Likewise, policies should be in place to insure that half-siblings, or others similarly related, do not unknowingly marry.

While the legal system has avoided interfering with reproductive choice, it has stayed away from making judgments regarding intimate family decisions, such as whether families created through donor insemination should disclose or not. It is possible that precedent has been established with adopted children, as the courts have required disclosure of information regarding their biological parents. Whether this will influence the courts regarding the psychological ramifications of donor insemination is unknown; however, if such issues become grist for the legal mill, there will be far-reaching implications for donors and the whole system of confidentiality. It may in fact discourage donors who do not want the possibility of identification or responsibility for a child thus conceived. And those on the other side, singles or couples who opt for donor insemination, will be equally affected, although in different ways. They may fear the potential interference of this stranger, but may possibly welcome some access that could provide ongoing information to their child.

Gay and lesbian singles and couples could use more assistance from the legal system. They have been affected more by moral than legal judgments and may benefit from increased legal intervention. For example, if a lesbian couple has a child through donor insemination, according to law both partners cannot be mothers. Therefore, the biological parent would have to relinquish her parental rights in order for the other to legally adopt the child (Keedle, 1994).

Surrogate Arrangements

Surrogate arrangements comprise another segment of the reproductive population that creates numerous ethical and legal entanglements. Although careful psychological screening of surrogates is usually required by medical institutions, it is not highly successful or accurate, judging from the number of court cases and extent of publicity. An agreement between the surrogate and the commissioning parents is drafted by a lawyer, but there are still questions about custody in numerous instances. For instance, when a woman carries a child conceived with donor sperm and her egg, she is still the genetic mother and therefore the legal mother. A significant distinction arises when a gestational surrogate is commissioned: Because she carries a child who bears no genetic connection to her, the court has decided in at least one case that the couple who provided the gametes and are the intended parents are the legal parents (Jaeger, 1996).

Other complications can occur if the surrogate desires to make decisions regarding the child or the pregnancy. She can, if she is genetically related to the embryo, terminate the pregnancy without the permission of the biological father (Herz, 1989). What about the complications that arise when the baby is defective or doesn't meet the parents' expectations? Who will care for the child? The legal significance of all of these potential complications are enormous. The social or emotional implications for the commissioning couple, the surrogate, her family, and the baby are psychologically overwhelming.

Embryo Cryopreservation

The cryopreservation of embryos has created another legal quagmire. It is predictable that some legal arguments would arise with donated embryos. That a couple might attempt to sue if a child is deformed or that the donating couple might renege on the agreement are understandable and even anticipated legal complications. What might not be anticipated, however, are potential custody battles over cryopreserved embryos. During a recent divorce, a couple disputed the fate of their preserved embryos. The trial court awarded custody to the wife and allowed her the option of implantation of these embryos (*Davis v. Davis,* 1989). In other cases, the courts have been called upon to make decisions regarding embryos from a deceased man, decisions about whether embryos can be transported beyond the borders of one country in order to seek medical assistance in another, and decisions about whether a couple can sue because the spouses did not achieve pregnancy with their own embryos when another couple was successful (Crockin, 1997). Although some of these cases represent problems arising in other cultures and countries, the implications are clear: Technology will forever challenge our legal imaginations and knowledge.

Genetic Engineering

Humankind has progressed from the genogram to the genome project. The jokes about clones are no longer jokes as biotechnicians move into engineering human life. What began as a government-sponsored international research and technical development effort is now feared as a method that could be used to create superbabies or a "super race."

The Human Genome Project was designed for the purpose of producing biological maps that could indicate all genes in the human body and determine the chemical sequence of DNA. Additional goals include developing programs and policies that address the ethical, legal, and social implications of obtaining such genetic information. Already, reproductive endocrinologists, fertility specialists, and other medical specialists are attempting to acquire the information obtained about genes (Blatt, 1996). What these specialists foresee is an ability to analyze the genetic material of the cells of donor gametes or embryos. This would then enable them to make a decision about using the donor prior to the genetic material being accepted. The positive aspect of this type of screening is the ability to avert implantation of a gamete that may carry a certain genetic disorder. Eventually, it may even be possible to manipulate the genetic material in order to delete the disease.

It is essential that medical and mental health professionals, legal experts, and consumers stay abreast of the developments in biotechnology and work to collectively shape the future of research and policy. In the excitement of such awesome developments, it can become easy to focus on "forseeing the cause" without adequately considering the possible ramifications. It is important that our society, and the larger international culture as well, do not allow new procedures to be used in ways that would discriminate against those with certain gene structures or problems. As with all potential reproductive technologies, vigilance is needed to insure equal access to the advantages such technology produces with commensurate responsibility to insure that the technology is used to promote health and well-being.

REFERENCES

Abbey, A., Andrews, F. M., & Halman, L. J. (1991). Gender's role in response to infertility. *Psychology of Women Quarterly, 15,* 295–316.

Annas, G. J., & Elias, S. (1989). The treatment of infertility: Legal and ethical concerns. *Clinical Obstetrics and Gynecology, 32,* 614–621.

Atwood, J. D., & Dobkin, S. (1992). Storm clouds are coming: Ways to help couples reconstruct the crisis of infertility. *Contemporary Family Therapy, 14,* 385–403.

Bader, E., & Pearson, P. T. (1988). *In quest of the mythical mate: A developmental approach to diagnosis and treatment in couples therapy.* New York: Brunner/Mazel.

Baluch, B., Al-Shawaf, T., & Craft, I. (1992). Prime factors for seeking infertility treatment amongst Iranian patients. *Psychological Reports, 71,* 265–266.

Baram, D., Tourtelot, E., Muechler, E., & Huang, K. (1988). Psychosocial adjustment following unsuccessful in vitro fertilization. *Journal of Psychosomatic Obstetrics and Gynecology, 9,* 181–190.

Barwin, B. N. (1993). Therapeutic donor insemination (TDI) for women without partners and lesbian couples: Considerations for physicians. *Canadian Journal of Human Sexuality, 2,* 175–178.

Berg, B. J., & Wilson, J. F. (1990). Psychiatric morbidity in the infertile population: Preconceptualization. *Fertility and Sterility, 53,* 654–661.

Berg, B. J., & Wilson, J. F. (1991). Psychological functioning across stages of treatment for infertility. *Journal of Behavioral Medicine, 14,* 11–26.

Berg, B. J., Wilson, J. F., & Weingartner, P. J. (1991). Psychological sequelae of infertility treatment: The role of gender and sex-role identification. *Social Science Medicine, 33,* 1071–1080.

Biddle, C., Roszia, S. K., & Silverstein, D. (1995). Kinship: Ties that bind. *Adoptive Families, 28,* 16–18.

Blatt, R. J. R. (1996). Conceiving the future: The impact of the human genome project on gamete donation. In M. H. Seibel, & S. L. Crockin (Eds.), *Family building through egg and sperm donation: Medical, legal, and ethical issues* (pp. 286–295). Sudbury, MA: Jones & Bartlett.

Bradt, J. O. (1989). Becoming parents: Families with young children. In B. Carter, & M. McGoldrick (Eds.), *The changing family life cycle: A framework for family therapy* (2nd ed., pp. 545–573). Boston: Allyn & Bacon.

Brown, L. S. (1995). Therapy with same-sex couples: An introduction. In N. S. Jacobson, & A. S. Gurman (Eds.), *Clinical handbook of couple therapy* (pp. 274–291). New York: Guilford.

Burns, L. H. (1990). An exploratory study of perceptions of parenting after infertility. *Family Systems Medicine, 8,* 177–189.

Burns, L. H. (1993). An overview of the psychology of infertility. *Psychological Issues in Infertility, 4,* 433–437.

Butler, R. R., & Koraleski, S. (1990). Infertility: A crisis with no resolution. *Journal of Mental Health Counseling, 12,* 151–163.

Callan, V. J., & Hennessey, J. F. (1989). Strategies for coping with infertility. *British Journal of Medical Psychology, 62,* 343–354.

Carter, B., & McGoldrick, M. (Eds.). (1989). *The changing family life cycle: A framework for family therapy* (2nd ed.). Boston: Allyn & Bacon.

Cole, D. (1988, March). Infertility tales. *Psychology Today,* 64–65.

Connecticut Women's Education and Legal Fund (1995). *The legal rights of lesbians and gay men in Connecticut.* Hartford, CT: Author.

Cook, E. P. (1987). Characteristics of the biopsychosocial crisis of infertility. *Journal of Counseling and Development, 65,* 465–469.

Cooper, S. L., & Glazer, E. S. (1994). *Beyond infertility: New paths to parenthood.* New York: Lexington.

Cramer, D. (1986). Gay parents and their children: A review of research and practical implicagions. *Journal of Counseling & Development, 64,* 504–507.

Crockin, S. L. (1997). Legally speaking. *ASRM News, 31,* 15–16.

Davis v. Davis, WL 140495 (1989).

DiNicola, V. (1997). *A stranger in the family: Culture, families, and therapy.* New York: Norton.

Dym, B., & Glenn, M. L. (1993). *Couples: Exploring and understanding the cycles of intimate relationships.* New York: HarperCollins.

Eck Menning, B. (1980). The emotional needs of infertile couples. *Fertility and Sterility, 34,* 313–319.

Eck Menning, B. (1984). The psychology of infertility. In J. Aiman (Ed.), *Infertility: Diagnosis and management* (pp. 17–29). New York: Springer-Verlag.

Eck Menning, B. (1988). *Infertility: A guide for the childless couple.* New York: Prentice Hall.

Erikson, E. (1950). *Childhood and society.* New York: Norton.

Erikson, E. (1964). *Insight and responsibility.* New York: Norton.

Floyd, C. C. (1981). Pregnancy after reproductive failure. *American Journal of Nursing, 11,* 2050–2053.

Freeman, E. W., Rickets, K., Tausig, J., Boxer, A., Mastroianni, Jr., L., & Tureck, R. W. (1987). Emotional and psychosocial factors in follow-up of women after IVF-ET treatment. *Acta Obstet Gynecol Scand, 66,* 517–521.

Fulmer, R. (1989). Lower-income and professional families: A comparison of structure and life cycle process. In B. Carter, & M. McGoldrick (Eds.), *The changing family life cycle: A framework for family therapy* (2nd ed., pp. 545–573). Boston: Allyn & Bacon.

REFERENCES

Gibbs, E. D. (1988). Psychosocial development of children raised by lesbian mothers: A review of research. *Women and Therapy, 8,* 65–75.

Glazer, E. S., & Cooper, S. L. (1988). *Without child: Experiencing and resolving infertility* (pp. 215–226). Lexington, MA: Lexington.

Gutman, M. A. (1985). Fertility management: Infertility, delayed childbearing and voluntary childlessness. In D. C. Goldberg (Ed.), *Contemporary marriage: Special issues in couples therapy.* Homewood, IL: Dorsey.

Halman, L. J., Oakley, D., & Lederman, R. (1995). Adaptation to pregnancy and motherhood among subfecund and fecund primiparous women. *Maternal-Child Nursing Journal, 23,* 90–100.

Harrison, K. L., Callan, V. J., & Hennessey, J. F. (1987). Stress and semen quality in an in vitro fertilization program. *Fertility and Sterility, 48,* 633.

Healy, D. L., Trounson, A. O., & Andersen, A. N. (1994). Female infertility: Causes and treatment. *Lancet, 343,* 1539.

Heiman, J. R., Epps, P. H., & Ellis, B. (1995). Treating sexual desire disorders in couples. In N. S. Jacobson, & A. S. Gurman (Eds.), *Clinical handbook of couple therapy* (pp. 471–495). New York: Guilford.

Herz, E. K. (1989). Infertility and bioethical issues of the new reproductive technologies. *Psychiatric Clinics of North America, 12,* 117–131.

Hindle, P. A. (1996). Charting uncharged waters: The role of the ethics advisory committee. In M. M. Seibel, & S. L. Crockin (Eds.), *Family building through egg and sperm donation* (pp. 219–223). Sudbury, MA: Jones & Bartlett.

Holbrook, S. M. (1990). Adoption, infertility, and the new reproductive technologies: Problems and prospects for social work and welfare policy. *Social Work, 35,* 333–337.

Imber-Black, E., & Roberts, J. (1992). *Rituals for our times: Celebrating, healing, and changing our lives and our relationships.* New York: HarperCollins.

In re Baby M, 217 N.J. Super. 313, 525 A.2d 1128 (1987), 109 N.J. 396, 537 A.2d 1227 (1988).

Jacob, M. C. (1995). Lesbian couples and therapeutic donor insemination. *Assisted Reproduction Reviews, 5,* 214–221.

Jacob, M. C. (1997). Concerns of single women and lesbian couples considering conception through assisted reproduction. In S. R. Leiblum (Ed.), *Infertility: Psychological issues & counseling strategies* (pp. 189–206). New York: John Wiley.

Jacob, M. C. (in press). Lesbian couples and single women. In L. H. Burns, & S. N. Covington (Eds.), *Infertility counseling: A handbook for clinicians* (pp. 1–28). New York: Parthenon.

Jaeger, A. S. (1996). Laws surrounding reproductive technologies. In M. M. Seibel, & S. I. Crockin (Eds.), *Family building through egg and sperm donation* (pp. 113–130). Sudbury, MA: Jones & Bartlett.

Kandrowitz, B. (1996, November 4). Gay families come out. *Newsweek, 51*–57.

Keedle, J. (1994, November 10–17). Bringing up baby: Gay and lesbian parents are redrawing the boundaries of the American family. *The Hartford Advocate,* pp. 14–18.

Kemeter, P. (1988). Studies on psychosomatic implications of infertility—effect of emotional stress on fertilization and implantation in in-vitro fertilization. *Human Reproduction, 10,* 323.

Kovacs, G. T., Mushin, D., Kane, H., & Baker, H. G. W. (1993). A controlled study of the psychosocial development of children conceived following insemination with donor semen. *Human Reproduction, 8,* 788–790.

Kübler-Ross, E. (1969). *On death and dying*. New York: Macmillan.

Laird, J. (1988). Women and ritual in family therapy. In E. Imber-Black, J. Roberts, & R. A. Whiting (Eds.), *Rituals in families and family therapy* (pp. 331–362). New York: Norton.

Leiblum, S. R. (1988). *Intimacy and the new reproductive options*. New York: Haworth.

Mahowald, M. B. (1996). Conceptual and ethical considerations in medically assisted reproduction. *Family building through egg and sperm donation* (pp. 262–273). Sudbury, MA: Jones & Bartlett.

Martin, A. (1993). *The lesbian and gay parenting handbook: Creating and raising our families*. HarperPerennial.

Matthews, R., & Matthews, A. M. (1986). Infertility and involuntary childlessness: The transition to nonparenthood. *Journal of Marriage and the Family, 48*, 641–649.

Mazure, C. M., & Greenfield, D. A. (1989). Psychological studies of in vitro fertilization/embryo transfer participants. *Journal of In Vitro Fertilization and Embryo Transfer, 6*, 242–255.

McCartney, C. F. (1985). Decision by single women to conceive by artificial donor insemination. *Journal of Psychosomatic Obstetrics and Gynecology, 4*, 321–328.

McDaniel, S. H., Hepworth, J., & Doherty, W. (1992). Medical family therapy with couples facing infertility. *The American Journal of Family Therapy, 20*, 101–122.

McEwan, K. L., Costello, C. G., & Taylor, P. J. (1987). Adjustment to infertility. *Journal of Abnormal Psychology, 96*, 108–116.

McGoldrick, M. (1989). The joining of families through marriage: The new couple. In B. Carter, & M. McGoldrick (Eds.), *The changing family life cycle: A framework for family therapy* (2nd ed., pp. 209–231). Boston: Allyn & Bacon.

McGoldrick, M., Pearce, J. K., & Giordano, J. (Eds.). (1982). *Ethnicity and family therapy*. New York: Guilford.

McGoldrick, M., Preto, N. G., Hines, P. M., & Lee, E. (1991). Ethnicity in family therapy. In A. S. Gurman, & D. P. Kniskern (Eds.), *Handbook of family therapy, Vol. II* (pp. 558–579). New York: Brunner/Mazel.

Mechaneck, R., Klein, E., & Kuppersmith, J. (1988). Single mothers by choice: A family alternative. In M. Braude (Ed.), *Women, power, & therapy: Issues for women*. New York: Haworth.

Melina, L. R. (1986). *Raising adopted children: A manual for adoptive parents*. New York: Harper & Row.

Mosher, W. D. (1988). Fecundity and infertility in the United States. *American Journal of Public Health, 78*, 181–182.

Muasher, S. J., Oehninger, S., Simonetti, S., Matta, S., Ellis, L. M., Liu H. C., Jones G. S., & Rosenwaks, Z. (1988). The value of basal and/or serum gonadotropin levels in prediction of simulation response and in vitro fertilization outcome. *Fertility and Sterility, 50*, 298.

Newton, C. R., & Houle, M. (1993). Gender differences in psychological response to infertility treatment. *Psychological Issues in Infertility, 4*, 545–559.

Nichols, W. C. (1988). *Marital therapy: An integrative approach*. New York: Guilford.

Pakizegi, B. (1990). Emerging family forms: Single mothers by choice—demographic and psychosocial variables. *Maternal-Child Nursing Journal, 19*, 1–19.

Parker, P. J. (1983). Motivation of surrogate mothers: Initial findings. *American Journal of Psychiatry, 140,* 117.

Parker, P. J. (1984). Surrogate motherhood, psychiatric screening and informed consent, baby selling, and public policy. *Bulletin of the American Academy of Psychiatry and the Law, 12,* 21.

Paulson, J. D., Haarmann, B. S., Salerno, R. L., & Asmar, P. (1988). An investigation of the relationship between emotional maladjustment and infertility. *Fertility and Sterility, 49,* 258.

Plows, C. W., & Howe, J. P. (1996). Issues of ethical conduct in assisted reproductive technology. *Joint report of the council on ethical and judicial affairs and council on scientific affairs,* Report A-96.

Robertson, J. A. (1983, October 28). Surrogate mothers: Not so novel after all. *The Hastings Center Report,* 34.

Sadler, A. G., & Syrop, C. H. (1987). The stress of infertility: Recommendations for assessment and intervention. In J. C. Hansen, & D. Rosenthal (Eds.), *Family stress* (pp. 1–17). Rockville, MD: Aspen.

Salzer, L. P. (1991). *Surviving infertility: A compassionate guide through the emotional crisis of infertility* (Rev. ed.). New York: HarperCollins.

Sandelowski, M. (1987). The color gray: Ambiguity and infertility. *IMAGE: Journal of Nursing Scholarship,* 70–74.

Scott, R. T., Jones, J. P., Muasher, S. J., Oehninger, S., Robinson, S., & Rosenwaks, Z. (1989). Follicle stimulating hormone levels on cycle day 3 are predictive of in vitro fertilization outcome. *Fertility and Sterility, 51,* 651.

Seibel, M. M., & Taymor, M. L. (1987). Emotional aspects of infertility. *Fertility and Sterility, 43,* 235.

Silverstein, R. (1995). Bending the conventional rules when treating the ultraorthodox in the group setting. *International Journal of Group Psychotherapy, 45,* 237–249.

Snarey, J. (1988, March). Men without children. *Psychology Today,* pp. 61–62.

Speroff, L., Glass, R. H., & Kase, N. G. (1994). *Clinical gynecologic endocrinology and infertility* (5th ed.). Baltimore: Wiliams & Wilkins.

Stanton, A. L., Tennen, H., Affleck, G., & Mendola, R. (1991). Cognitive appraisal and adjustment to infertility. *Women & Health, 17,* 1–15.

Statistical abstracts of the U.S. (1987). Washington, DC: U.S. Government Printing Office.

Stewart, D. E., & Robinson, G. E. (1989). Infertility by choice or by nature. *Canadian Journal of Psychiatry, 34,* 866–871.

Stovall, N. W., Tomah, S. K., Hammond, M. G., & Talbert, L. M. (1991). The effect of age on female fecundity. *Obstetrics & Gynecology, 77,* 33–36.

Tauer, L. N. (1996). The costs of single parent adoption. *Adoptive Families, 29,* 56–57.

Todd, T. C. (1986). Structural-strategic marital therapy. In N. S. Jacobson, & A. S. Gurman (Eds.), *Clinical handbook of marital therapy* (pp. 71–105). New York: Guilford.

United States v. Jacobson, 785 F. Supp. 563 (E. D. Va. 1992).

Valentine, D. P. (1986). Psychological impact of infertility: Identifying issues and needs. *Social Work in Health Care, 11,* 61–69.

Whiting, R. A. (1988). Therapeutic rituals with families with adopted members. In E. Imber-Black, J. Roberts, & R. A. Whiting (Eds.), *Rituals in families and family therapy* (pp. 211–229). New York: Norton.

Williams, L., Bischoff, R., & Ludes, J. (1992). A biopsychosocial model for treating infertility. *Contemporary Family Therapy, 14,* 309–322.

Wright, J., Allard, M., Lecours, A., & Sabourin, S. (1989). Psychosocial distress and infertility: A review of controlled research. *International Journal of Fertility, 34,* 126–142.

Zoldbrod, A. P. (1993). *Men, women and infertility: Intervention and treatment strategies.* New York: Lexington.

INDEX